Tourette Syndrome

Stop Your Tics by Learning What Triggers Them

TOURETTE SYNDROME
STOP YOUR TICS
BY LEARNING WHAT
TRIGGERS THEM

SHEILA ROGERS DEMARE

ASSOCIATION FOR COMPREHENSIVE NEUROTHERAPY

Grosse Ile, Michigan

www.Latitudes.org

Published by the Association for Comprehensive NeuroTherapy (ACN)
P.O. Box 159, Grosse Ile, MI 48138-0159, USA

Disclaimer: The material in this book is for educational purposes only, and is not intended as specific treatment recommendations for individuals or as medical advice. The suggestions in this book are not intended as a substitute for consulting with a physician. No product, practice, or practitioner mentioned in this book is being endorsed. Neither the editor, the Association for Comprehensive NeuroTherapy and its board members, *Latitudes.org* and its professional advisory board, nor any related party, make any claims regarding the effects of the therapies and approaches discussed; they cannot accept legal responsibility for any approach or treatment undertaken. Please consult a qualified health care practitioner for appropriate treatment.

Rogers DeMare, Sheila
Tourette Syndrome: Stop Your Tics by Learning What Triggers Them

For information and correspondence please address the author:
Sheila Rogers DeMare, Director ACN, P.O. Box 159, Grosse Ile, MI 48138-0159, USA
Contact: acn@Latitudes.org

ISBN: 978-0-9763909-2-3

*This book is dedicated to everyone who takes the
initiative to explore triggers for tics and shares
their findings for the benefit of others.*

Acknowledgments

I would like to thank Larry Teich for his valuable insights and contributions to this text. Special thanks to physicians Joseph Rogers, Felix Rogers, and Bob Moore for their professional recommendations.

Jan Fenner's dedicated attention to detail, and Helaine Sutton's assistance in finalizing the book, are appreciated. Steven Polyanchek's graphic skills and clear vision of our organization's mission proved invaluable in completing this project. I am grateful to my daughters Mona and Rose, to whom I often turn for advice, for ongoing feedback and support. Thanks also to Sandy Glassman and Tana McLane for their design consultations.

I would also like to express thanks to my sister, Dr. Lisa Rogers. A neuro-oncologist, she has been a steady source of encouragement and a thoughtful "sounding board" since the start of my efforts in this field.

I especially owe a deep and heartfelt debt of gratitude to Christopher Grayson for his manuscript advice and for keeping me on track throughout this process—an effort which proved to be no small task.

And to my husband Frank: My apologies for the extended time I spent working on this book. Your support has made all the difference (even if you did turn my mantra "I'm almost done" into a punchline). You are the best.

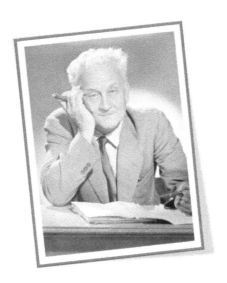

"Discovery consists of seeing what everybody has seen, and thinking what nobody has thought."

Albert Szent Györgyi
1937 Nobel Laureate in
Physiology and Medicine

Contents

SECTION ONE

The number of people dealing with tics has skyrocketed over the last few decades. In this chapter you will learn about the three main types of tics being experienced, and which conventional efforts are being used to control symptoms. Find out what triggers are, and why most people do not know about allergic, dietary, and environmental triggers for tics, even though an awareness of them could change their lives for the better.

It is common practice for doctors to discuss triggers for certain medical conditions with their patients. For example, heat can cause hives, excessive caffeine can trigger a seizure, paint thinner fumes can cause a migraine, and a virus or spicy foods might trigger a flare-up of Crohn's disease in someone with the condition. Knowing about potential triggers gives patients a starting point when exploring factors that may be affecting their symptoms. Read how this applies to tics.

When you repeatedly witness that a certain food, toxin, scent or allergen aggravates tics, you know the connection is real. This is the case regardless of what your doctor or the medical literature says based on conventional thought. When triggers are removed and tics consistently improve, you have an increased motivation to continue with your efforts. My young son's amazing recovery from Tourette syndrome is shared here with the hope that it helps advance the understanding and treatment of tic conditions.

SECTION TWO

SECTION THREE

SECTION FOUR

11 After identifying triggers 121

The goal of a trigger search is to identify problems so you can avoid them in the future. Figuring out the triggers is one thing—avoiding them is something else! Use suggestions in this chapter to get a better handle on this important phase in your efforts.

SECTION FIVE

12 Get help: Trigger-Resources webpages 129

We have created several free tools to help with your trigger investigations. Whether you are exploring this area for yourself or for a loved one, having relevant links, practitioner information, logs for adults and teens, and incentive charts for use with children can make a positive difference in your efforts. Details on the special web resource pages, developed as a supplement to this book, are given.

13 How you can help this effort 161

Please see our list in this chapter of ways you can help spread the word about triggers for tics and Tourette's. We need your support to strengthen this vital message, promote research, and increase the impact of the work of our nonprofit organization.

SECTION SIX

Letter from the author

The serious tic disorder known as Tourette syndrome was recently described in a professional publication as one of the "most mysterious medical curiosities on the planet." And, we are told, "the causes of abnormal twitches and movements remain completely unknown."[1]

This sobering assessment comes after more than 40 years of advocacy and ongoing study of tic conditions.

Another status update is provided by the 2015 1st World Congress on Tics and Tourette's. The document concludes: "*The management of Tourette syndrome is challenging and has remained largely unsatisfactory through the last decade of intensifying clinical and scientific interest in the condition.*"[2]

Given that experts consider the causes of Tourette's to be baffling, and that current treatment management is acknowledged to be unsatisfactory, the public should expect that no stone would be left unturned in an urgent search for new answers to tic conditions. Yet, this has not been the approach in this field.

From the same World Congress report noted above, we read that genetics are estimated to account for 60% of Tourette syndrome risk, and that "other, non-genetic (environmental) factors are also very important in the development of this disorder." This is not a new finding, but this collaborative statement makes it clear that the medical community needs to look beyond genetics for answers.

To date, the primary research emphasis for tic disorders in general, and Tourette's in particular, has overwhelmingly focused on genetics, along with disappointing attempts to find suitable drug therapies. Meanwhile, for decades, patients, families, and integrative physicians have reported that they have noticed and documented an association between tics and allergic, dietary, and environmental triggers.

Triggers—which can cause or increase symptoms—play a key role in many medical conditions, and through this book I propose that tic disorders are no exception. The encouraging fact is that the identification and avoidance of tic triggers has the potential to improve symptoms, along with or without the use of standard or other integrative approaches.

The time has come for the public to be fully advised on what is currently known about triggers for tics, and for international studies to begin.

If you or someone you care about is dealing with a tic disorder, it is my hope that this book encourages you to go beyond standard medical advice and explore what may be initiating or exacerbating tic symptoms. While answers are not always easy to find, and no approach applies to everyone, when triggers are identified and avoided, positive change can be right around the corner.

The Association for Comprehensive NeuroTherapy (ACN: *Latitudes.org*), a nonprofit organization, is the lead group focusing on the issue of triggers for tics and Tourette syndrome. As founder and director ACN, I invite others to join forces in defining this important area.

Sheila Rogers DeMare
Director, Association for
Comprehensive NeuroTherapy
www.Latitudes.org

Introduction

The value of being aware of symptom triggers

Imagine a panicked father rushing his daughter to the emergency room every time she has a life-threatening asthma attack. How would he feel to learn, many years later, that exposures to sulfite preservatives in foods, or cat dander, or smoke from his home fireplace might have triggered some of these attacks? He would surely wonder how many traumatic crises could have been avoided if he had been aware of potential triggers for his child's asthma.

Or, think of a mother whose son suffered painful migraines for years. This mom would understandably be upset to one day discover that certain favorite foods she served had triggered some of his headaches. We can picture her frustration: "Why didn't someone tell me this could happen?"

Fortunately, these scenarios are not as likely today as they were 20 years ago. Standard medical protocols for treating asthma and migraine now include the topic of environmental, dietary, and allergic triggers. In fact, a quick internet search yields multiple lists on mainstream medical websites detailing potential triggers for both asthma and migraine. Yet, there is no such information widely shared about triggers for tics.

Now imagine you are the parent of a young boy who developed serious symptoms of Tourette syndrome—a tic disorder with both verbal and motor (movement) tics. The child is anxious and upset about his ongoing jerks, twitches, and uncontrollable vocalizations. He repeatedly begs you to help, to make the tics go away. You would do anything you could to make them disappear, to restore calm and confidence to your child. But you do not know what to do. Actually, you have been told by doctors that there is not much you *can* do!

Then, one day, you learn that the food you are putting on the family break-fast table is making your child's tics worse for the rest of the day. You find that certain personal products are triggering symptoms, that the orange Gatorade® at soccer practice sets tics off, and exposures to common aller-gens are aggravating the tics. And that is just for starters.

This was our family's experience. How did I feel when I saw this firsthand? I was frustrated not to have known that tics could be affected in this way. But, I was also grateful to have a chance to begin helping my child by nailing down triggers and eliminating as many as we could. It was not long before we had the symptoms under control with the help of an integrative allergist who focused not just on allergy therapy and nutritional balancing for my child, but on a range of allergic and environmental triggers, including diet, that can affect the nervous system. I share our family's story in Chapter 3.

Four goals for this book are to:

- Increase awareness of allergic and environmental influences that have the potential to affect tics.

- Provide specific trigger lists and tools to aid in determining personal triggers.

- Encourage avoidance of triggers.

- Highlight the need for research into triggers for tics and Tourette syndrome, and encourage funding for new efforts that focus on this area.

Section One

Tics and triggers: The basics

The importance of trigger lists

The gift of discovering triggers: My story

Allergic, dietary, and environmental impacts on tics

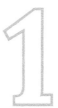

Tics and triggers: The basics

Types of tic disorders

Tics are involuntary and repetitive movements or vocalizations that tend to be sudden and rapid. Movements, also referred to as "motor tics," as well as vocalizations (see examples below) can be simple or complex in nature, and can range from mild to severe.

A few examples of the many ways tics might be expressed:

Examples of simple motor tics: neck jerks, eye blinking, nose twitches, shoulder shrugs, lip biting, muscle tensing, jaw snapping, tongue thrusting, eye rolling

Examples of complex motor tics: twirling or jumping, skipping, hopping, imitating someone's actions, chewing clothes, twirling hair, obscene gestures, and smelling or touching something. Also, self-injurious behaviors like touching hot or sharp items, hitting self

Examples of simple vocal tics: a light cough or throat clearing, repetitive humming, grunting, a loud shout, a yelp or bark, hissing, snorts, squeals or screams, tongue clicking, gasping

Examples of complex vocal tics: calling out words, repeating one's own words (palilalia) or other people's words (echolalia), or the use of obscene words (coprolalia), and talking to self

Vocal tics can interrupt the smooth flow of a normal conversation, or they can occur at the beginning of a sentence much like a stutter or a stammer.

People often feel a sensory urge to tic, and many report that they can temporarily postpone some tics. After ticcing, there is usually a sensation of released tension. Tics might be so minimal that they are barely noticed, or so intense that they are physically painful or damaging to the body, disruptive to daily life, and/or emotionally distressing. Some tics are more socially unacceptable or embarrassing than others.

Three main types of tic conditions are defined in the latest edition of the *Diagnostic and Statistical Manual of Mental Disorders* (DSM-5): Provisional tic disorder; Persistent (chronic) motor or vocal tic disorder; Tourette syndrome.[3]

Please note that these categories are used by physicians and psychologists to provide a diagnostic label for tic symptoms. There is no lab or imaging test to identify or differentiate tic disorders. Each has its own specifications, yet the symptoms are more similar than they are different.

Conditions in the bulleted list below apply to all three tic conditions, according to the DSM-5. Specific criteria for each type follows:

- Tics should have started before the age of 18. They may wax and wane in frequency;
- They should not be due to taking medicine or other drugs, nor due to a medical condition (for example, Huntington disease or post-viral encephalitis).

A *provisional tic disorder*: Single or multiple motor and/or vocal tics. The tics have been present for less than one year.

Persistent (chronic) motor or vocal tic disorder: Single or multiple motor or vocal tics have been present—but not both motor and vocal. The tics have persisted for more than one year.

Tourette syndrome: Both multiple motor and one or more vocal tics have been present at some time, although not necessarily concurrently. The tics have persisted for more than one year.

Research specific to Tourette syndrome is noted as such in this book. Otherwise, the terms "tic disorders" or "tic conditions" are used as general terms to include the three categories just described. Also, "Tourette's" is often used in this text as an abbreviated term for Tourette syndrome.

A range of medical conditions can be associated with tics—such as a thyroid disorder, restless leg syndrome, bacterial or viral infections, Lyme disease, dystonias (uncontrollable muscle contractions), or seizures. For that reason, consultation with a neurologist or other qualified physician is recommended for a definitive diagnosis of tic symptoms. When major bouts of tics start up suddenly, it is important to consider causes, such as an adverse reaction to medications, or a toxic exposure, or an infection (such as strep, as one example).

The number of people with tics has been increasing

Researchers often comment in their publications that prevalence rates for tics and Tourette syndrome are "higher than previously thought." That is an understated way of pointing out that tic disorders are spiking.

The number of people with tics conditions, including Tourette's, has been rapidly increasing for decades. Dr. Kevin Black reported in 2016 that for transient (also known as provisional) tics: "Prevalence depends strongly on age, with the highest rate probably about 20% at age 5–10. Lifetime prevalence is much higher . . . The available evidence supports the view that tics occur at some time or another in a large fraction of all children, probably over half."[4]

While estimates vary, Tourette syndrome is reported to occur in up to 1 in 100 children.[5] The rate is highest in special education classes. The diagnosis of Tourette's is twice as likely in non-Hispanic white persons as in Blacks or Hispanics. Approximately three times as many males as females experience Tourette symptoms.[6]

Once rare, Tourette's is now considered to be a common condition, and experiencing transient tics is very common.

Most cases of tics are mild, in which case the symptoms may not interfere with a person's lifestyle, and medical treatment may not be sought or needed.

Reportedly, by age 18, half of children who previously had tics may be tic-free, with some others showing improvement. However, patient reports of symptom improvement can be subjective, and it has been suggested by Dr. E. J. Pappert that many adults report being tic-free when they actually still have tics. In Pappert's study, videotapes of adults with Tourette syndrome were compared to videos of the same people when they were kids. It was found that, while the tic severity had decreased by adulthood in this group, about 50% of those who thought they were tic-free did, in fact, still have tics.[7]

Conventional approaches to tics

Unfortunately, progress in defining genes for Tourette syndrome has proven very difficult, although some rare genetic mutations have been documented. Research is intensifying in this area, with coordinated global efforts. Neuroimaging has detected some structural or metabolic changes in the brain for some people with Tourette's, but these findings have not yet resulted in successful targeted treatments to reduce tic symptoms.

Due, in part, to the lack of clarity regarding the causes of tics, it is difficult for practitioners to know which medication might be best suited for a given patient. Determining the most effective drug that carries the least negative reaction is often a trial and error process, and responses can be very patient-specific. With this in mind, doctors often start with a low dose of a medication and increase it gradually, in an attempt to minimize adverse responses.

Another confounding issue when prescribing drugs for tics is that 80-90% of people with Tourette syndrome also have one or more coexisting conditions, such as attention deficit hyperactivity disorder (ADHD), obsessive compulsive disorder (OCD), anxiety, sleep problems, depression, and/or other medical issues.[8]

New efforts are continually underway to discover better therapies, with medications at times prescribed off-label (not approved by the FDA for a particular use). Drugs that are often considered for treating significant tic symptoms include typical and atypical antipsychotics, anti-seizure medications, medicine for high blood pressure, and botulinum (Botox) injections.

Some people take themselves off prescribed drugs, or refuse to take them in the first place, due to concerns over potentially serious side effects and lack of sufficient effectiveness. That said, medication can often provide some measure of relief from tics.[9]

For severely affected patients with disabling tic symptoms who have not responded to medications, deep brain stimulation, via electrodes surgically implanted in the brain, is being used as an option. Obviously, this invasive procedure carries risks. In a 2014 study led by Dr. J. Zhang, outcomes for this technique were reviewed. Results showed that the Gilles de la Tourette Syndrome-Quality of Life Scale score improved by approximately 50% after a period of 2 to 3 years of deep brain stimulation treatment.[10]

Integrative approaches to tics

The current lack of safe and effective therapies for tics has resulted in an ever-increasing focus on non-drug approaches. Behavioral therapies are one such field. Comprehensive behavioral intervention for tics (CBIT) has been shown to reduce tic symptoms by training patients to become aware of their tics, having them engage in competing behaviors when they feel the urge to tic, and changing daily activities to avoid situations that lead to ticcing.

CBIT, which is growing in popularity, does not help everyone reduce tics, but no single approach does. It requires ongoing awareness and effort by the patient, with ten or more training sessions usually needed. Generally, children below the age of ten are not yet aware of having urges to tic, so they are not ideal candidates for CBIT. Plans are underway to increase the number of providers.[11] Other promising related techniques, such as habit reversal therapy, have also been used to reduce or change the way tics are expressed.

Additional integrative approaches pursued by patients and families seeking relief from tics include biomedical interventions that address underlying physiological imbalances, nutritional therapy, detoxification, allergic and immune modifications, acupuncture, dental appliances, diet management, trigger identification and avoidance, and neurofeedback or biofeedback. Each of these approaches is addressed in our organization's book *Natural Treatments for Tics & Tourette's: A Patient and Family Guide.*[12] We hope that needed research will begin in these areas in the near future.

What is a tic trigger?

A trigger is anything that initiates symptoms or makes them worse. Note that these influences are rarely the underlying cause of a medical condition. For example, strobe lights are a recognized trigger for seizures in someone with photosensitive epilepsy. The lights are not the actual underlying cause of this condition, but exposure to them has the potential to induce a seizure in a susceptible person. Avoiding strobe lights does not mean that the person no longer has epilepsy. But avoidance of this trigger can improve the quality of life by reducing symptoms.

While there is often an overlap among influences to which people with tics react, triggers need to be determined at an individual level. What bothers one person may not affect someone else. One person may be hypersensitive to a multitude of factors, while another might find just one or two issues to be particularly problematic. Some people may not be aware of any triggers.

The search for tic triggers can be well worth the effort, and lifestyle changes to address them often bring about a positive change in symptoms.

The types of daily triggers discussed in this book are not the same as the issues commonly considered to be environmental "risk factors." This text focuses on day-to-day influences and exposures that might aggravate someone's tics. In contrast, risk factors studied for Tourette's, to date, include issues like prenatal and perinatal events. For example: maternal stress or weight gain, depression, anxiety, smoking, use of cannabis or alcohol, infection during pregnancy, socio-economic status, and low birth weight.[13-16] These represent prior conditions over which patients have no control.

Why most patients do not know about triggers for tics

Many are not familiar with the concept of tic triggers beyond issues like stress, fatigue, anxiety, and excitement, all of which are often reported by the tic community. Clinicians rarely discuss a variety of potential dietary, environmental, or allergic triggers. In fact, families often tell me that when they asked doctors whether these influences might affect tics, the clinicians discouraged them from exploring these issues, even specifying it would be "a waste of time" to do so. Then, if the patient or parent reported having already noticed that there was a connection between tic symptoms and diet, allergens, and/or chemical exposures, they were usually instructed that this must have been a coincidence, that they were surely mistaken.

It would appear that these physicians, understandably, take their lead from the medical literature and mainstream advocacy organizations. Neither of these sources currently shares information on tic triggers. Further, a bias against dietary tic triggers has been observed in research (see pages 20-22).

I should point out that practicing physicians are not universally adverse to the concept of triggers. After all, they recognize them for a number of medical conditions (see page 17). Rather, most are simply not yet aware of the range of potential triggers for tics.

Why have triggers for tics and Tourette syndrome been ignored? It is hard to say, but one reason is a long-standing, almost exclusive emphasis on the role of genetics in these disorders. The standard advice to patients dealing with Tourette's is that it is a "hereditary condition for which there is no cure." Patients are typically told that they should expect tics to spontaneously come and go on their own. The term for this so-called unavoidable pattern is "waxing and waning."

Tics are said to be mysteriously waxing when they worsen, and waning when they improve. But what if this waxing is due to a trigger that could have been avoided—something in one's diet or environment, a sensory experience, or an allergic response? If so, it would naturally be helpful to be aware of these potential influences so they could be watched for, addressed, and, when feasible, avoided. You can learn a great deal about personal triggers through your own observations, as well as by working with a qualified health professional who understands this approach.

The bottom line

Tics are experienced worldwide by many millions of people of all ages. Whether tics are serious enough to dramatically impair the quality of life, or so mild as to be barely noticeable, they have no redeeming value. They are a symptom that should be addressed, and they should not be considered normal or inconsequential just because they are now very common.

To date, researchers do not have good answers to explain why, during recent decades, there has been a significant upswing in the number of people experiencing tics. With this book I propose that until triggers for tics are thoroughly examined, the troubling increase in tic prevalence will not be fully explained.

As often pointed out in this text, triggers are person-specific. What bothers one person may not affect someone else. Further, not everyone may be able to identify their tic triggers. However, when they can do so, there is new and valuable opportunity for symptom improvement.

Notes

The importance of trigger lists

The potential for environmental, dietary, and allergic triggers to modify symptoms of specific medical conditions is well-established. There is a long-standing practice of compiling lists of possible triggers based on feedback from patients, and from family members when a child is involved. Typically, self-reports form the basis for trigger exploration.

**Some of the many medical conditions
or events with recognized symptom triggers**

ADD and ADHD	Fibromyagia
Anaphylaxis	GERD
Anxiety	Hay fever
Arthritis/Gout	Headache
Asthma	Hives
Atrial fibrillation	Irritable bowel syndrome
Autism	Lupus
Colitis	Migraine
COPD	PANDAS/PANS
Crohn's disease	Parkinson's disease
Depression	Psoriasis
Eczema	Rosacea
Epilepsy	Trigeminal neuralgia
Essential tremor	Ulcerative colitis

Physicians often instruct patients with tics that symptoms will appear and disappear for no known reason. As a result, people naturally feel disempowered (not to mention frightened), and they are less likely to consider looking for an associated cause-and-effect connection with symptoms.

Trigger lists for tics serve an important purpose in opening people's minds to the possibility that they may actually have some degree of control over their symptoms. Such lists also increase public understanding of the potential role of allergy, diet, and the immediate environment in triggering or exacerbating tics. Beyond this, of course, items on trigger lists give examples of specific factors for people to consider and monitor.

Identifying and avoiding triggers is a useful and practical part of an integrative approach to the treatment of tic disorders. Results of a self-report survey on tic triggers by ACN (*Latitudes.org*) are shown in Chapter 7. This survey was completed by nearly 2,000 people. The results have been updated to include additional reports received online from around the world, as well as triggers shared by participants at Tourette syndrome conferences.

Potential triggers are just that: items or exposures that might trigger or worsen a symptom in someone with a given condition. No list applies to everyone. At the same time, no list of trigger possibilities can be considered exhaustive. In other words, someone may find they react to something that is not included on trigger lists.

Pushback on tic trigger information

I have been told by some Tourette syndrome advocates that information on triggers should not be provided to the public because it might get people's hopes up, and "studies do not support it." I would agree that there is a dearth of research on tic triggers. But it is misleading to assert that studies do not support something, implying that research refutes the concept, when actually, very little research on the topic has been undertaken. Most trigger lists are developed based on personal feedback provided through reports and surveys rather than on formal studies for specific trigger items. Such research is not a requirement before information can be ethically shared.

As for "getting people's hopes up," if fail-proof therapies, only, were endorsed in the field of medicine, no approaches would be offered. Is all information on cancer therapies, or weight-loss methods, or cardiac procedures withheld simply because the interventions will not be successful with everyone?

There is no presumption by ACN (*Latitudes.org*) that everyone with tics has the same tic triggers, nor even that everyone has identifiable triggers. The point is that they do exist, and people have the right to know this.

One of the most irresponsible comments we hear from mainstream voices is along these lines: "If indeed there is a connection between tics and diet or environmental issues, it is experienced by only a small subset of people." This claim is fabricated, because studies have not looked at this issue. The claim is made in an effort to downplay the importance of this topic.

A failure by advocates to promote common sense

Sometimes research on a specific trigger is conducted, and depending on the circumstances, this approach can be useful. But it should not be a prerequisite for alerting the tic community about possible influences that may affect symptoms.

As an example, increases in tics have been reported to ACN (*Latitudes.org*) after an exposure to pesticides. Obviously, it would be unethical to purposely expose people to these agents, which are already known to be toxic to the nervous system, just to study how different age groups of people with tics react, or how long an exacerbation continues. Rather, it is common sense that exposures to products designed to disrupt the nervous system should be avoided by people with Tourette's and tics. Reports received from people who have inadvertently been exposed to pesticides and experienced tics as a result reinforce this.

This is not to say that the global roles of pesticides and herbicides as underlying causes of tic disorders should not be vigorously investigated, as has occurred with Parkinson's disease. Such an effort is needed. But people dealing with tics need to be made aware *now* of the potential for these harmful products to aggravate and stress the nervous system. Children are particularly vulnerable.

Regarding other types of triggers, when multiple people report symptom increases from consuming particular foods, or after being exposed to allergens, or from encountering chemicals like those used in treated swimming pools or cleaning materials, there is no ethical reason to withhold these findings from the public. After all, people can decide for themselves if they wish to explore trigger possibilities. But first, they need to know that triggers exist.

To date, our organization's completed survey is the only large-scale effort to explore triggers for Tourette's and other tic conditions. ACN (*Latitudes.org*) welcomes feedback from related studies on a range of dietary, allergic, and environmental triggers. During the last fifteen years, the Tourette Association of America (operating as the Tourette Syndrome Association at the time) conducted two surveys on non-drug approaches to tics. Dietary factors, nutrient supplementation, and allergy were among the topics included. The results of these surveys have never been released to the public.

Blatant research bias against dietary tic triggers

It is particularly concerning when researchers exhibit bias against dietary tic triggers in the course of a study. The only relatively large published study on Tourette's and diet is from Germany: "The influence of different food and drink on tics in Tourette syndrome." Among 224 survey respondents, almost half (47%) reported that coke (cola) worsened tics in themselves or children, while 34% said coffee did. Black tea was also a trigger. And, a significant percentage responded that 1) preserving agents; 2) refined white sugar; and 3) sweeteners worsened tics.

Note: Based on the journal article, artificial colors and flavors were excluded from the list of survey items that respondents could choose from. Yet, the authors acknowledge that in research by others, coloring has been proven to trigger hyperactivity and behavioral change.

The study conclusion stated that only caffeine affects tics. The fact that colas, the greatest offenders, typically have less caffeine than coffee, while containing sugar, corn syrup, or artificial sweeteners, plus synthetic coloring, preservatives, and/or added flavoring, was ignored. Also, the separate finding that preserving agents, white sugar, and sweeteners were reported to increase tics was dismissed. The authors say they could not understand how these items could affect tics, so they omitted these responses from their conclusion.

The convoluted reasoning for burying these results was: "Since it is general knowledge that preserving agents and white sugar in excess is unhealthy, the consumption of these foods, therefore, might gnaw at one's conscience, thus might cause stress and this, in turn, might deteriorate tics." Further, it was suggested that since these items are thought to affect ADHD symptoms, participants may have "generalized the negative attributes of these foods." Finally, the researchers could not explain why a significant number found that a sugar-free diet was helpful, so those responses were also deemed irrelevant.

It appears the researchers preferred to psychoanalyze the thought process of survey respondents rather than acknowledge that their findings did not support their study hypothesis: "Nutrition does not influence tics in patients with Tourette syndrome."

This spin on survey results is far-fetched and unsettling. Why not accept all survey responses received? New findings are an opportunity for fresh discoveries in a field that desperately needs them. And, why conduct a survey on food and drink in the first place if you are not prepared to believe the observations of the tic community? The conclusion in the journal report, emphasizing that only caffeine should be considered an aggravating factor in tics, did not even call for additional study.

Ironically, in the article the authors say that they find it "remarkable" that not many reported using a special diet as an approach to tics. Yet, *this journal article is a perfect example of why most people do not consider changing their diets!* The report unfortunately promotes the false belief that food and drink do not play a role in tics. It misleads and disempowers patients and families, and it discourages future research.

The conclusion should have included wording like this:

> *In addition to caffeine, for reasons not understood by the investigators, unidentified ingredients in cola, as well as preservatives, white sugar, and sweeteners, may exacerbate tics in a subset of patients. Additional research on food and drink in tics in Tourette's is warranted.*

Müller-Vahl, Kirsten R., Nadine Buddensiek, Menedimos Geomelas, and Hinderk M. Emrich. "The Influence of Different Food and Drink on Tics in Tourette Syndrome." Acta Paediatrica 97, no. 4 (2008), 442-446.

Taking a cue from migraine trigger research

Based on reports provided to ACN (*Latitudes.org*), perfume is a potential allergic trigger for tics. What follows is one of my favorite trigger reports:

> Many of us with Tourette's have a "punny" sense of humor. My mind is always looking for any chance for some word-play. I read in publications by your organization that perfumes and scented products can

> be triggers for tics. I already knew that a strong perfume scent could aggravate my tics.
>
> I am a clerk at a Canadian post office, and one night I was sorting bundles of magazines entitled *Cosmetics*. I was looking at this title word on cover after cover. Then my Tourettic mind started looking at it from a different angle. I saw the title become "cos-me-tics," pronounced "cause me tics." And it's true—they can cos me tics!

This gentleman made his own discovery that perfumed products trigger his tics. When he learned that our publications reported the same, he was inspired to offer his story. We are grateful that he shared his observations with us in hopes that others would learn of this tic response as well. But we should ask ourselves: Why was he left to discover this reaction on his own instead of through standard literature on tics?

Perfume is a researched, documented trigger for migraine. This is of special interest because there is a fourfold increase in the incidence of headache and migraine among children and adolescents with Tourette syndrome (Ghosh 2012).[17] Given this connection, it is only logical that some of the research efforts for migraine and headache are also relevant to tic conditions.

As of June 2017, there were fifteen published research studies on perfume as a trigger for migraine.[18,19] Yet, there is not even one study on tics or Tourette's and perfume. That said, perfume is only one of many items that can negatively impact the nervous system and potentially cause, or trigger, tics.

In the next chapter I explain why promoting awareness of tic triggers has been a focus of my life for more than twenty-five years.

Notes

3

The gift of discovering triggers: My story

My 8-year-old son's symptoms of vocal and motor tics developed gradually. During the coming year, I watched helplessly as symptoms changed from simply being troublesome to creating emotional, social, and physical distress. Dealing with the tics, which were accompanied by uncharacteristic mood swings, began to consume my family's days.

First it was eye rolling and winking, then persistent shoulder shrugs. Strong neck jerks came next, followed by occasional full-body tics. He also had vocal tics and developed some self-injurious behaviors. After trying to conceal or control the tics at school, he would return home in a hyperstressed state. Compounding all this were obsessions that seemed to have emerged from nowhere. My boy's social life began to suffer, and self-esteem bottomed out.

If a mother's tears could have cured him, I would not be writing this book. I was a single parent in Florida with three kids, working full-time as a school psychologist, and desperately wanting to help my child.

We consulted a neurologist who was highly recommended for dealing with tic disorders. After making the diagnosis of Tourette's in my son, the doctor told us that the condition is genetic and there is no cure. He advised that medications could be used, but he warned against their side effects.

We should be aware, he said, that the tics will come and go on their own, and the term for this is waxing and waning. He added with a smile that I am sure was meant to be comforting: "No one ever died from Tourette syndrome."

We returned home from the clinic feeling more frustrated and hopeless than when we had arrived. A no-cure label applied to my child's symptoms was of little use. I needed to know what I could do to truly help my son.

The turning point

I wondered: How could a happy-go-lucky, terrific kid now have an out-of-control body that was impacting so much of his life? Why was this happening, and was I just supposed to accept it? The entire situation did not make sense. I began searching for alternative approaches, which was not an easy task in the 1990s. Little was available online, so I scoured books and literature.

The most accessible information was on drug therapy, and after reading about their side effects, I knew they would need to be a last resort.

Meanwhile, symptoms worsened. One day I was at home when my son came through the front door with major motor and vocal tics. He was in extreme distress; the symptoms were much worse than usual. He went to his bedroom to be alone, and just then the phone rang. It was my sister, a neurologist, calling long-distance. When I heard her voice I burst into tears. I simply could not bear watching my son tormented in this way. She knew we had already consulted a specialist, and she calmly said, "You never know, Sheila. Maybe someday you will be able to help other people who are dealing with Tourette's." Nothing could have seemed more unlikely.

When the school year came to a close and summer break began, we drove to a small condo on the west coast of Florida for a week's vacation. I told my son and his two older sisters that we were going to celebrate school being out, and they should enjoy themselves. I gave them permission to spend lots of time in the community pool, and to walk to a nearby convenience store for a treat each day. I also lightened up with meals, allowing more "fun" items than I usually would.

Surely the tics would be better, I thought. My son could now relax, with no peer pressure or school work. Yet, to my surprise the symptoms were worse. I was heartsick and confused.

It was hot and humid when we stopped at a motel for an overnight stay on the drive home. After checking in, I called for maintenance because the air conditioner was not working in our musty-smelling room. We watched in disgust as the repair man removed a vent cover from the ceiling and thick globs of discolored slime cascaded down in long strands. He matter-of-factly stated the obvious, telling us that the vent needed cleaning. We left the room so he could work on it, and came back later to sleep.

That evening I watched my boy as he stretched out on top of the bed and closed his eyes. He looked so sweet in his summer shorts, his skin tanned after a week in the sun. But I was soon dismayed. For the first time, his entire body was in spasm. His arms, legs, and back all had little twitches coming and going. I instinctively dropped to my knees with a desperate prayer—a prayer that when I took my child back to the doctor for the drugs that we could no longer avoid, he would still be able to function and have a happy life.

Moving in a new direction

Once back home and before connecting with our neurologist, I fortunately heard from another mother in Florida, Ginger Wakem. She had started an informal alternative therapy network, with the goal of sharing information about an allergy connection to tics. Ginger told me about a doctor who had reversed her son's severe case of Tourette's. I made an appointment right away. Now retired, Dr. Albert Robbins, an allergist and environmental physician, provided specialized allergy therapy for my son and also taught us about food reactions, nutritional imbalances, and chemical sensitivities. I will forever be grateful to both Ginger and Dr. Robbins. For the first time, I had new hope for my child.

We learned how the immune system, the environment, diet, and allergy can affect the nervous system and the brain, triggering tics. When these types of issues were addressed, tic symptoms disappeared, along with the behavioral and emotional concerns. When we were lax, issues began to resurface, at which time we would quickly tighten up our efforts. Within a few weeks, there was observable improvement and we knew we were on the right track. Within six months, a devastating condition had been brought well under control. We were thrilled with the results.

Putting it all together

Prior to this experience, I did not know people could react negatively to low levels of common toxins like cleaning products and scented items. I had no idea that sugars, certain foods, allergens, and synthetic additives could affect behavior and aggravate tics. I did not know that the health of the digestive system was connected to the functioning of the brain and nervous system.

If someone had asked me before this healing if I had ever noticed triggers for either my son's tics or his behavioral changes, I would have said no. I never knew to look! In fact I was not even aware that he was allergic. Neither his pediatrician nor his neurologist ever brought up the possibility.

I thought back to our tic-filled vacation week. The things I had assumed were great ideas—lots of time swimming in the (chlorinated) pool, and being able to enjoy junk-food treats that were not usually allowed at home—were in fact harmful for him. And, the experience at the musty motel allowed me to see firsthand how a mold exposure could affect the nervous system and cause muscle spasms. It was a real eye-opener, but only in retrospect. Plus, had the exposure not been so major, so glaring, I do not think I would have made the association between mold and tics.

Here is just some of what I learned over the first few months of this new approach:

- A number of foods and drinks were clearly making tics worse.
- My son had a systemic candida overgrowth that was affecting digestion.
- I was unaware he had a dust allergy, and dust control measures were needed.
- Insect bites increased tics temporarily.
- Exposure to scented personal products and strong cleansers increased tics.
- A mold allergy was affecting symptoms.
- He had a major reaction to standard pesticide products, like bug spray.
- Specialized allergy therapy was needed, with nutritional deficiencies treated.

Efforts to spread the word: ACN begins

Like most in the Tourette community, I had believed that my child's tics were inevitable and out of our control. A new world had now opened up for us. The treatment for my son was a complete success, and medications were never needed.

Without a doubt, the recovery was not a coincidence, nor did he "outgrow" the problem. His body was healed. While nutritional balancing and a specialized allergy treatment were important parts of his therapy, identifying and avoiding triggers played a critical role. If we had overlooked his triggers, full recovery would not have been possible.

One day, I learned that the national Tourette Syndrome Association (now the Tourette Association of America) had received reports of successful natural therapies for tics, and descriptions of tic triggers, for many years before our family's struggles began. Yet, the public was not aware of these reports. I began serving as a volunteer liaison to this association's medical advisory board at their request. After several years, it was clear that I was unable to bring about change, unable to get them to widen their view of underlying causes of Tourette syndrome. They showed no interest in exploring dietary, allergic, and environmental connections to tics, and we ended the liaison connection.

I recall the chairman of the board at that time suggesting to me that I was misguided, that my son would have recovered anyway, spontaneously. My response was: "It is rather offensive to be told that I did not see something that I very clearly saw." Much of my son's suffering and our family's distress could have been avoided if we had known about the possibility of different types of triggers.

Tic disorders can impact all aspects of life, from achievement and careers to relationships, family life, self-esteem, and personal goals—not to mention physical well-being. It is not enough for advocacy organizations to spend millions of dollars every year raising awareness, sharing strategies for coping with tics, giving educational support to families and school staff, and striving to reduce bullying. These are all noble efforts. But families and patients need to know everything they can possibly do to reduce symptoms, and this includes being aware of potential triggers.

Eventually, Ginger Wakem requested that I take the lead with her alternative therapy effort. I developed a newsletter with an advisory board comprised of leading specialists in integrative medicine, and in 1996 I founded the 501(c)3 nonprofit Association for Comprehensive NeuroTherapy (ACN). The website *Latitudes.org* followed. I wanted to spread the message that the treatment of tic disorders should include a "comprehensive" range of integrative approaches. Other neurological conditions, including ADHD, OCD, autism, behavior and learning problems, PANDAS/PANS (see pages 114-116), and depression are among the focus of our organization.

We are encouraged by the growth of our nonprofit association and the positive response we have received to our efforts. We are also pleased that our book, *Natural Treatments for Tics & Tourette's: A Patient and Family Guide*, has often been the Amazon bestseller on the topic of Tourette syndrome over the past several years. It is the only comprehensive guide on how to treat tics, twitches, and related neurological conditions using a variety of natural and alternative or integrative therapies. More recently, ACN launched *StopTicsToday.org* to raise much needed funds for research.

Notes

_____

_____

_____

_____

_____

_____

_____

_____

_____

_____

_____

_____

_____

_____

_____

_____

_____

Allergic, dietary, and environmental impacts on tics

There is a saying: "Genetics loads the gun and the environment pulls the trigger." A classic way to explain how the environment can affect tics focuses on identical twins. Both will have the same genes and presumably the same predisposition for developing, for example, tic disorders. Yet studies show that the degree of symptom involvement can vary widely between twins, due to different experiences and conditions that begin in the womb and continue throughout life.

Recent research advancements focus on epigenetics, the study of how genes can be affected by the environment. The "environment" includes physical, chemical, biological, dietary, and social impacts on health, which can all influence how genes are expressed.

From the standpoint of a medical discipline known as environmental medicine, a health issue like tics is looked at as a problem that needs to be explored or investigated, not as something that should be accepted with resignation. The environment impacts you every day of your life. While some environmental effects are beyond our control, other influences can be addressed, often with positive results.

What a person eats, drinks, touches, and smells or inhales, along with issues like infection, hormones, thoughts, emotions, and stress, are all types of environmental influences. If you do not examine the possible causes for symptoms, you cannot hope to fully address healing.

The goal of an environmental medical evaluation is to:

- Determine what previous exposures or conditions may have resulted in a person's health complaints.

- Treat any underlying issues.

- Identify ongoing triggering factors that may be playing a role in the development or aggravation of symptoms.

- Encourage avoidance of offending triggers.

Author and neurologist David Perlmutter, MD, maintains that we are exposed to neurotoxins every day that can damage brain and nerve cells. In *The Better Brain Book*, he identifies the six most concerning toxins for the brain and nervous system as: pesticides, mercury, aluminum, lead, excitotoxins (food additives), and electromagnetic frequencies.[20]

Key environmental factors in health

- Parental health; prenatal, birth, and postnatal conditions
- Food and drink
- Pathogens
- Drugs
- Odors, fragrances
- Allergens: pollens, dust, molds, animals
- Seasons, temperature change
- Indoor environments
- Stress, thoughts, emotions
- Sensory input

- Radiation, including electromagnetic forces
- Toxins, including toxic metals and chemicals

Do not overlook the obvious

Many doctors are not aware of the role of the environment in health, and they fail to consider it. Medical students in the U.S. receive minimal training on how to recognize and manage environmentally-related diseases. If they were well trained in this concept, environmental influences would be more readily identified and causes of health effects would be more obvious, allowing for better prevention and treatment.[21, 22]

Anything can seem like a mystery if it is not carefully examined. When tics worsen, something is causing that. When tics are better, something has allowed that to occur. The challenge is to uncover which factors are involved and deal with them as best as possible.

Dr. Leo Galland wrote in *The Allergy Solution* (2016): "Nothing produces such dramatic relief as identifying an allergic trigger and eliminating it."[23]

Research on allergy and intolerance in Tourette's

While studies on tics and allergies are scarce, those conducted over the past 20 years confirm a connection to allergy. The research is summarized below.

1) In a conference paper presented at the 20th Congress of International Association of Child and Adolescent Psychiatry & Allied Professions in Paris (2012), Dr. Koray Karabekiroglu wrote that his team found that OCD and tic disorders have a "robust association" with allergic diseases in children and adolescents.

2) In 2014 Dr. M. Yuce reported that a preliminary study showed an association between allergic diseases and Tourette's and/or OCD.[24]

3) Researchers for Tourette's have identified a gene that disrupts histamine production. Histamine is both a neurotransmitter and an immune modulator. Cacabelos and co-workers noted in 2016 that mice given this mutated gene began to experience symptoms consistent with Tourette's.[25]

4) Additional studies have also confirmed a connection with tics and allergy, including one led by Dr. C. Ho in 1999: "The prevalence of allergy in Tourette syndrome patients in our study was significantly higher than in the general population. Tourette syndrome had an association with allergy." [26]

5) Further, Yu-Tzu Chang and others indicated in 2011: "Our data showed significant correlation between allergic diseases and Tourette syndrome. Risk also increased with the number of allergic comorbidities and with age."[27]

While these findings do not imply that everyone has an allergic or immune connection to their tic condition, those dealing with tics should consider this possibility. Further research should be pursued by the scientific community.

First reports: Diet, the environment, and tics are linked

The immune or allergy connection to Tourette syndrome was first identified by Theron Randolph, MD, in the 1950s. His efforts were expanded upon in the late 1970s by Marshall Mandell, MD. An allergist, Mandell spent more than one thousand hours at his own expense in a search for causes and triggers for tics.

Through his clinical work with patients, Dr. Mandell observed a significant link between allergy and Tourette's. Aware that the condition was viewed as a mysterious and incurable genetic disorder, he was excited by his findings. He took the opportunity to share his observations at an international medical conference on Tourette syndrome—with no response from participants. Also without success, he tried to convince mainstream advocacy groups that treating allergy and controlling for triggers like diet, mold, inhalants, and chemical exposures could help reduce tic symptoms.

Dr. Mandell continued his efforts to spread the word about the tic-allergy connection by serving as a valued member of our organization's volunteer advisory board until his passing. He was an unsung hero in the search for answers to tics. Subsequent to his findings, many other physicians, families, and patients followed his lead, investigating allergy and triggers for tics, and often successfully reducing symptoms.

One of the first written parent accounts of allergy, chemicals, and dietary triggers for Tourette syndrome was provided by a cardiologist. He sent his letter to the Tourette Association of America (Tourette Syndrome Association) in the early 1980s. Included below, his letter was initially shared in a flier by the association but was removed from their literature list many years ago. I have published it before and do so again, because the father's observations are insightful and worthy of respect. He wrote, in part:

> Although my daughter never displayed any typical allergy symptoms, it was found that she is allergic to many foods, some molds and pollens, and is highly sensitive to chemicals. She was placed on a rotation diet. She has been on the diet for four months and is being desensitized to molds and pollen. I have eliminated as many chemicals as possible from her food and environment.
>
> Her reduction in tics while on the diet was 85%. I took her off the diet while she was on a trip with another family. Within two days, her tics significantly increased, and within one week, they dramatically increased. By dramatic, I mean nonstop tics with several vocalizations, as opposed to one simple tic every one to two minutes, and very slight, if any, vocalizations. Emotional and intellectual patterns that I had not necessarily associated with Tourette's also reappeared at this time.
>
> I observed her reaction to chemicals. With each exposure, her tics would double. An exposure to fluorides doubled her tics for two days. An expo-

> sure to a diesel motor running in front of our home increased her tics the entire period the motor ran. An exposure to paint doubled her tics for six hours. An exposure to paraffin in a small restaurant with many burning candles produced nonstop tics until we left the restaurant.
>
> In my opinion, her sensitivity to chemicals produces a marked increase in the intensity and frequency of her symptoms.

This physician-father was able to connect the dots between his daughter's tic increases and her exposures to certain foods, allergens, and chemicals. He took the "mystery" out of her symptoms.

In the late 1980s, Dr. Doris Rapp, a board certified pediatric allergist, appeared on the *Phil Donahue* show and described an allergic component in Tourette's. Accompanied by patients and parents, she explained how foods and chemicals could impact tics and behavior. The families involved verified that they had seen tic symptom improvement with allergy treatment and the avoidance of triggers. The program received a major public response. Yet, Dr. Rapp told me during a personal conversation that she was never contacted by any professionals in an effort to learn more about the successful approach she used.

Throughout her career, Dr. Rapp often videotaped patients in her office to demonstrate reactions to allergic and environmental exposures. It was an effort to convince skeptics that exposure to toxins, allergens, and foods could affect a person's nervous system, learning, and behavior. Invariably, she complained, the patients in the videos were accused of acting. Frustrated, she eventually gave up trying to convince the medical community and instead continued her practice and wrote international best-sellers on the topic. Her classic text, *Is This Your Child? Discovering and Treating Unrecognized Allergies in Children and Adults*, was published in 1991 and has a chapter on Tourette's. It was followed by *Our Toxic World: A Wake Up Call.*

Retired from practice, Dr. Rapp is now in her 80s and still advocating for awareness of environmental health issues. As an aside, I was scheduled to be the keynote speaker at a 2016 national Tourette syndrome conference. I contacted her to ask if she had any special advice for me. Her response was: "Yeah. Give 'em hell." (*Note to Dr. Rapp*: I did my best. I doubt I will be invited back.)

Food allergy and intolerance

Dr. J. R. Gerrard published an interesting report in 1994 on the role of diet in movement disorders.[28] The work of Gerrard and his co-workers showed that "episodic movement disorders" could be triggered by foods or components in the diet. He reportedly videotaped the reactions and wrote, in part:

> In the first patient, the movement consisted of shaking the head from side-to-side. That was triggered by milk and a number of other foods.

> In the second patient, the movement consisted of a repeated shrugging of the shoulders triggered by egg and coffee.

> In the third, the movement consisted of rhythmic contractions of the arms and legs that were triggered by aspartame (i.e., Nutrasweet; Equal).

The authors concluded:

> These observations suggest that, in susceptible individuals, foods can trigger movement disorders through an action on dopamine and other neurotransmitter pathways in the brain.

I mention this report for a few reasons. First, it supports the feedback received by ACN (*Latitudes.org*) documenting that a variety of foods and drinks have the potential to trigger motor tics. Second, it shows that reactions can be patient-specific. Third, this was published more than 20 years ago, and follow-up studies are clearly needed.

Food reactions: a complex issue

Food allergy and food intolerance, or sensitivity, are topics of controversy among allergists. This controversy applies to both assessment and treatment approaches. A full discussion is beyond the scope of this book, yet this simplified summary by Dr. Albert Robbins addresses some of the key issues of this complex subject:

Some forms of "food intolerance" are not considered food allergy, even though symptoms may be similar. True "food allergy" is immune-mediated.

Immediate reactivity or *IgE mediated food allergy*: This is a "fixed" food allergy and is usually inherited, meaning genetically determined. These foods may need to be completely removed from the diet or avoided if symptoms are serious. This is referred to as Type 1 IgE-mediated food allergy. Allergy immunotherapy can help in some cases.

Delayed reactivity or hidden food allergy is IgG-mediated: This is a cumulative type of allergy. The body develops antibodies against foods eaten frequently. Many chronic illnesses triggered by food allergy are associated with delayed or cumulative food allergy.

Sometimes a food allergy is a concomitant allergy. A concomitant food allergy might be related to a pollen or mold allergy. This is a masked or hidden food allergy. For example, in hay fever season, certain foods, such as milk, melons, or bananas, should be avoided if you are allergic to ragweed.

It is important to note that the scientific medical literature supports the viewpoint that food allergy is often an overlooked cause or aggravating factor in chronic illnesses. Yet, many physicians do not consider food allergy as a cause of illness. When food allergy is discovered and properly treated, it sometimes prevents the need for symptom-relieving medication.

Allergy testing is not always going to give you the full picture on sensitivities. There are a number of reasons for this, including the fact that different types of allergists use different methods of testing. The gold standard for food allergy/sensitivity detection is to completely avoid all foods containing a specific suspected item (such as milk or corn) for a period of four to seven days. This is called a single-food elimination diet. Then, after the elimination, you plan to eat a significant amount of the food during a one-day period and watch for reactions. In some cases it is advisable to do this test in the presence of a physician in case a severe response occurs.

Another approach is to use a multiple-food elimination diet for which you remove several foods to which people are often intolerant, and monitor for a change in health, emotions, or behavior. Then, add them back one by one and watch for reactions.

Detailed plans on elimination diets are usually available from an allergist, nutritionist, or integrative physician, and, of course, in books on the subject. It is best to have a plan developed, with needed foods on hand, before beginning the diet.

Dr. Jonathan Brostoff, an international expert on food sensitivities, suggests that if a food you are intolerant of is avoided for an extended period, you may be able to consume it again as long as you do not over do it. (This process does not apply to food allergies.) He recommends that for the greatest relief from food reactions, it is important to avoid everything you may be sensitive to at the same time. He cautions that removing only one food from the diet while still eating or drinking other troublesome items may not help you track down food culprits. His book, *Food Allergies and Food Intolerance: The Complete Guide to Identification and Treatment* is highly recommended for a comprehensive explanation of how to determine and treat food sensitivities. Updated in 2000, it is a classic text.

What foods are most likely to cause problems?

There is so much diversity in immunological responses to diet that any list of common items can only be considered a starting point.

Foods commonly known to cause any number of different physical reactions are, in alphabetical order, beans, beef, chocolate, citrus, coffee, corn, dairy milk, eggs, fish, grains (especially gluten-containing), peanut, potato, shellfish, soy, and tree nuts. However, immune responses can occur from a wide range of unadulterated natural foods, as well as prepared food and drink products. In addition to particular foods, synthetic additives including flavorings, preservatives, colorings, and certain artificial sweeteners can be troublesome.

Studies have yet to define which foods are most likely to affect tics versus those causing other types of reactions, such as hives, breathing problems, difficulty swallowing, digestive complaints, or low blood pressure, to name just a few.

A list of foods reported by patients and families as triggering tics are included in Chapter 7, with anecdotal reports provided in Chapter 5. These reports should be considered preliminary.

Some may find that foods with a high glycemic index can aggravate tics by increasing the blood glucose level, or by negatively affecting the balance of bacteria in the digestive tract. Both of these situations can result in the nervous system being more reactive, with an increase in tics.

What percentage of tic patients are affected by diet?

It would be useful to know the percentage of people with tic disorders who experience an increase in symptoms after consuming certain foods and beverages, but there is presently no research that addresses this.

The role of diet in neurological health tends to be a hotly debated topic. Once substantial research begins on diet and Tourette syndrome, it will no doubt be many years before a consensus is achieved within the medical community.

As an example of what can be required for a consensus, beginning in the 1950s, literally *hundreds* of studies have been published on diet triggers for headache and migraine. Yet, I was surprised to read a review of this topic in the *Journal of Head and Face Pain* by Drs. Martin and Vij (2016). It begins: "The role of diet in the treatment of headache disorders is one of the most controversial topics in the field of headache medicine."[29]

At issue is not whether food and drink can trigger headaches. That is a given. But, defining the triggers, determining which are the most prevalent (and for which subgroups), and being able to recommend a diet to avoid triggering a headache or migraine, are all ongoing challenges.

The subject of dietary tic triggers should not be avoided by the medical community simply because it may be complex, and because it would move the field into new frontiers.

While the tic community waits for studies, it should at least be common knowledge that diet can indeed affect both motor and vocal tics. People need to have the option of exploring whether this connection applies to their case or not.

Gluten or wheat sensitivity with or without celiac disease

Gluten, a protein found in wheat, rye, and barley, is a documented tic trigger for some people. Among those who notice a tic problem with gluten are an unknown percentage with celiac disease, as well as some others who have tested negative for the condition. People are sometimes confused when they notice they seem to feel better when they do not consume gluten or wheat, yet they do not have a diagnosis of celiac disease or wheat allergy.

Celiac disease is a serious autoimmune disorder that occurs in genetically predisposed people. For these individuals, the consumption of gluten leads to damage in the small intestine. It is estimated to affect 1 in 100 people worldwide. When someone with celiac disease eats gluten, their body mounts an immune response that attacks the small intestine. These attacks lead to damage on the villi, the small finger-like projections that line the small intestine. When the villi get damaged, nutrients cannot be absorbed properly. People with a first-degree relative with celiac disease have a 1 in 10 risk of developing celiac disease. (Source: *Celiac.org*)

Laboratory tests to diagnosis celiac disease include a blood test for gluten autoantibodies and a small bowel biopsy to assess gut damage. (For accurate results, the patient needs to be consuming gluten prior to testing.)

Self-reports of gluten sensitivity by people with neither celiac disease nor wheat allergy are on the rise. This problem is now considered an emerging medical condition. "Non-celiac gluten sensitivity," referred to as NCGS, and "non-celiac wheat sensitivity" (NCWS), are receiving scientific scrutiny after patient complaints were dismissed for many years.

One or more symptoms that may resolve when removing gluten (or just wheat) from the diet of people with these sensitivities include tics, depression, a "foggy-head," hyperactivity, bloating, diarrhea, abdominal pain, joint pain, and fatigue, among others.

A significant increase in the number of people wishing to avoid gluten has led to the development and marketing of many "gluten-free" items now featured online and in special sections of grocery stores. In the West, restaurants have started to adapt their menus to include gluten-free offerings.

Dr. Luis Rodrigo, a researcher at Central University Hospital of Asturias in Oviedo, Spain, shared with me in late 2016 that he is following more than fifty cases of people with a diagnosis of Tourette syndrome who do not have celiac disease, but who have benefited from a gluten-free diet. According to Dr. Rodrigo, his findings include the observations that at times improvement in tic symptoms is gradual, and that in some instances other foods are also found to be involved and need to be avoided. He does not suggest that gluten is a problem for all Tourette patients, but says that it can be an important issue for some.

Only an elimination diet, or trial and error, can confirm or refute a problem with gluten among non-celiac persons.

Section Two

Advice from the tic community

5

Advice from the tic community

This chapter features excerpts from letters selected from many received by ACN (*Latitudes.org*). While included here for their variety, you will note some overlapping of triggers among writers. Most of these reports are newly shared; some were also published in our book *Natural Treatments for Tics and Tourette's* or can be read on our website. In total, they represent a snapshot of the types of experiences people have had in exploring tic triggers. Numerous health care professionals have reported similar findings.

These letters were written by people who ignored the standard belief that there was little they could do on their own to reduce tics. They explored a variety of influences and, once successful, shared their findings to help others. To provide anonymity, actual names of authors are not used.

A heartbreaking report: an adult discovers his triggers

The first account highlights portions of a report from a man with Tourette's who did not discover his major, life-changing triggers until he was an adult. By this time, his severe symptoms had caused great suffering to himself and his family. I hope readers will reflect on how different life could have been for him if information on tic triggers had been general knowledge when he was growing up, and if his family had known to look into potential triggers. Although other family members were not formally diagnosed, the writer believes he has a family history of Tourette syndrome.

PATRICK: A friend sent an email containing articles by your group about patients with Tourette syndrome, with a link to your website *Latitudes. org*. I wanted to share some things I have discovered by experimentation and close observation of my Tourette symptoms through the years.

I'm a 49-year-old Caucasian male, and I have been experiencing Tourette's constantly, in varying degrees, throughout my life since its onset at age seven.

Life was difficult in primary school, and the tormenting I received from the other children in response to my facial tics, head-shaking, grunts, and "hooting" sounds prevented me from having any close relationships or making even casual friends. In high school, dating seemed impossible, as my self-esteem was further eroded.

My father still remembers me shaking my head so violently that he thought I would break my neck or throw myself out of a chair. He felt so powerless to do anything to help me that he cried.

I had an EEG during one especially severe bout of tics but the results were inconclusive. No neurological or regional brain centers appeared to be specifically involved. After I had fallen asleep [during testing], the alpha and theta waves were normal. A doctor prescribed Thorazine and later Haldol. These medications made me sleepy, and I could not stay awake in school. Tics were somewhat reduced, by perhaps 40% at best, but I was unable to perform; I slept a great deal of the time.

I focused on my primary interests of science and engineering. After I taught myself to play rock guitar I was "socially accepted" at parties or social gatherings. They were usually trivial friendships at best, but at least my social status was greatly improved.

My grades were never all that good, and the medications just made things worse. I eventually dropped out of high school during 12th grade. High school academics had became unbearable for me. College was totally out of the question.

My tics were fairly constant, but occasionally became quite severe through my early 20s, especially during periods of great stress.

As the years passed, I began noticing the things that appeared to either worsen or improve my tics, or more precisely, my "urges" to tic. The anxiety and tension around this urge to tic was actually more bothersome than the tics themselves. I learned to "defer" some tics by conscious effort. Example: I would flex muscles in my legs instead of shaking my head or making facial tics.

One day at work, I noticed that soon after eating cold cut meats in my lunch sandwich, an intense and rapid onset of head-shaking and vocal tics occurred. I had run out of money for lunches that week, and so I had resorted to making my lunch at home. Lunch meats, bread, cheese, and mayonnaise were on my home "menu," but with disastrous results.

I wondered why I had never noticed this happening before and concluded that I must have been experiencing a quiet and low point in my tics, thus making this more noticeable. I decided to make these same sandwiches for lunch over a two-week period as an experiment.

After the third day, I was experiencing tics that were totally out of my control, even with my new technique of deferring tics. The tics lasted throughout the day and into the evenings. These were head-shaking and facial tics, with some percentage of vocalized noises.

I was basically working alone during this period, so that made things easier. After the two-week period, the tics had reached a high and constant level that changed very little. I then stopped using the cold cuts and other lunch meats in my sandwiches.

After having purposely triggered intense tics for two straight weeks, the symptoms were slow to subside, but gradually the tics, urges to tic, and the associated anxiety were greatly reduced.

After about two months I had no outwardly noticeable tics. They had been reduced to the usual nominal level. And, after a few more weeks, the tension and anxiety involving the urge to tic was reduced to such a low level that hours would pass without my even thinking about it.

Later I had only temporary increases in tension and tics due to stress (when laid off from my job) and a lack of at least six hours of quality sleep.

A few months later, I attended an electronics symposium at which breakfast was being served. I had bacon, eggs, and hash browns with toast and coffee for my breakfast. Soon after eating the breakfast, I experienced a sudden (and I mean sudden!) onset of tics of the head, face and neck. These came on within half an hour of the breakfast. I was unable to control the tics with any notable success. I suspected the bacon, largely because of my awareness of the high degree of preservatives and coloring agents used in the manufacturing of most bacon. The tics subsided by the next morning.

At the next symposium breakfast, I had exactly the same meal—the same amounts of all the same foods, except I skipped the bacon. I finished the breakfast and noticed there was no increase in the tension or urge to tic. In fact, I had several cups of caffeinated coffee that morning, and even a chocolate bar after lunch that day, just as I'd had the previous day when I had consumed the bacon. I should add here that I have never noticed any change in my tics or tensions resulting from consuming coffee, tea, chocolate of any kind, or even alcohol and cigarettes. Only the nominal—what I call the "noise floor" level of tics and urges—were observed all that day.

I was very interested in what the bacon and lunch cold cuts had in common. I began reading packages of various brands of these products. I discovered that they all contained various amounts of sodium phosphate, sodium erythorbate, and/or sodium nitrate(s). Seemingly every brand had these compounds added to their processed meats. I was obviously sensitive to these chemical additives.

To date, the above are the most significant observations I've made about the severity of my motor tics and their frequency as related to foods, stress, and lack of sleep.

I suggest that readers who suffer from tics and Tourette's be conscious of what they eat, and read the labels of food products, especially processed and preserved meats, and canned goods. I encourage experimentation with foods and other factors that alter or modify a person's tics, tensions, and anxiety—and keeping good records.

A *comment by the author on the previous report*

In addition to highlighting the importance of investigating triggers, this account is a good example of how individualistic tic triggers can be. This man did not notice a major increase in tic levels from consuming chocolate, coffee, or alcohol–or even from smoking–yet some people dealing with tics have reported one or more of these to be quite troublesome.

Of course, any of these items may have contributed to the daily "noise floor" level of symptoms he mentioned. But in his case, it was chemical additives in foods, specifically nitrates, that he found caused severe tic reactions. (Similar products without nitrates or additives are increasingly available. Check all labels carefully.)

Other personal accounts are included in this chapter. Throughout the book, pages for notes are provided for you to document any topics that resonate as possible issues for you and your situation.

Wheat and additives as culprits

SANDRA: Several months ago we started to look for food intolerance in our seven-year-old son. Since that time we have come to realize that certain things cause him to have particular tics.

Artificial colors (particularly tartrazine yellow and red dyes) plus artificial flavors and most preservatives are troublesome. These seem to affect eye blinking, eye rolling, and sighing; and they change his breathing patterns. They can also alter his demeanor, making him wild, reckless, easily frustrated, and sometimes slightly aggressive. They can cause a lack of concentration and make him argumentative all-around; he's just not himself. So we avoid these.

Wheat is a major problem for him, causing near constant coughing tics, throat-clearing, and other vocal tics. Since removing all wheat and substituting white rice flour or another alternative, and avoiding additives as mentioned, he is now virtually tic-free. Be aware of hidden wheat, because it is everywhere!

We are continuing to watch closely, but by simply staying as close to natural as possible, making our own breads, muffins, and snacks while avoiding wheat, we have seen a huge change, as have close family members who are now trying to support him by having wheat-free snacks on hand, and not being so quick to offer treats. Thank you for having a forum on *Latitudes.org* to support what could be an overwhelming task. It gives parents a place to start!

An adult recalls his childhood tic triggers

JONATHAN: As a kid, I had a diagnosis of Tourette syndrome for several months before my family learned that toxins and allergies were a big part of my problem. I was in elementary school and had a lot of neck jerking, eye wincing, and shoulder tics. Plus, I had vocal tics. My family tried to hide how worried they were, but I could see it was hard for them, not just for me. Along with this, I started to get obsessions and anxieties that I never had before.

After going to a few doctors and getting diagnosed with Tourette's, we learned by trial and error that artificial flavors and colors could make me hyper and cause tics. Tics would usually start up shortly after I ate foods with these things in them. I would often also experience "foggy headed-ness" based on the types of foods that I ate.

I didn't always want to believe that some of my favorite foods were affecting me. For example, I remember cinnamon raisin bread being a real trigger, more than plain bread. Was it the cinnamon or the raisins or something else? I don't know, but I stopped eating it even though I liked it. Once I was sure something was a problem, I gave it up as best I could. Of course I experimented at times, but I would usually pay a price (this included drinking alcohol in college).

When I swam in a pool that had chlorine or other chemicals, both of my eyes would start to roll a lot. For that, I cut back on the time I spent swimming, and would wear goggles while in the pool and shower right afterward. This helped lessen the reaction.

Strong smelling shampoos, soaps, and cologne could also make my tics worse. We bought unscented natural products, not just for me to use but for the whole family. This also included cleaning and laundry supplies. When I experimented it was very clear that chemicals could trigger my tics, just like foods could.

I feel very blessed that my family was able to help me identify my tic triggers at such a young age. Not only did the dietary and environmental changes drastically reduce my tics, but the changes also encouraged me to adopt a healthy lifestyle. I'm a married adult now and doing really well, aside from some mild hay fever. I watch what I eat and I take nutritional supplements. My wife and I make sure the home doesn't have any toxic chemicals or typical scented products such as air fresheners or candles. She even gave up her favorite perfume for me. I have been symptom-free for many years, but I still avoid all additives in foods, and eat organic and non-GMO when I can. I minimize sugar intake, and am always on the alert for anything that might aggravate my nervous system.

Multiple food triggers

STEVEN: Neither growing up with a chronic tic disorder myself nor having a brother with Tourette syndrome prepared me for the day when my young son began showing signs of Tourette's. My wife and I noticed that tics worsened after ingestion of dairy products and corn chips (with no apparent reaction to blue corn). Upon RAST blood testing, he was found to be allergic to milk, corn, oats, and certain fish. After restricting the offending allergens from his diet, we observed a 99% reduction in tics. The only tic remaining was a verbal murmur in the mornings and evenings. After putting a HEPA air purifier in the house, the verbal tics disappeared.

Today, my son is tic-free unless he eats something in school that sets him off. He also has undergone a complete change in disposition. He no longer gets overly frustrated, and he's happier more of the time. His behavior in school has also improved. The medical profession tends to dismiss such success as spontaneous remission. I know that is not the case, because I can reproduce the tics by introducing the offending allergens back into his diet.

Our success did not come easily, but has been well worth the effort. I recommend to other parents that once you know you're on the right track, do not give up. If you run into a setback, do more investigating, keep looking, and chances are you'll find you have missed something.

Video and TV as triggers

RACHEL: We are in the beginning stages of more aggressively looking for food triggers, but the most obvious problems for our seven-year-old son are video games and TV, especially in a dim room, and the computer. His tics increase tenfold. He is aware of this himself and is willing to drastically limit

TV. He has given up video games and limits computer time desperately wants some control over his tics.

As parents it is at times completely overwhelming, especially, younger siblings, but we are all committed to aiding our son in his search for answers to Tourette syndrome. Making him an active participant and having a lot of open dialogue about possible causes has helped him, and that in itself seems to have decreased his tics.

He has bouts on return from school and can be cranky and confrontational due to the effort and stress of suppressing his tics, so we try to give him quiet time to de-stress and then have a family physical activity like take a walk, go for a bike ride, etc.

If he is willing to try, who are we to not give him every opportunity?

In support of all parents and children in the same situation, keep faith, and persevere. Take it at any pace but continue to move, search, and grow in your knowledge.

Our successful search for problem foods

JORGE: My 8-year-old had severe, disabling tics for several years. At their worst, they would stop him from doing homework and feeding himself because he couldn't control his hands. Sometimes he couldn't speak because he had to go through a 15-second routine first. He was often on the verge of tears and it was absolutely gut-wrenching for all of us.

The tics ran from sucking in his stomach, to mouth-stretching, to hand-stretching, neck-stretching, vocal tics, swallowing repeatedly, and also ADHD symptoms that went with it.

I have been through health issues of my own, and was helped by seeing a local dietitian and getting a food intolerance test. Since my son seemed to have frequent stomach pain and nausea, and there definitely seemed to be a food connection, I decided to have him tested for both allergies and food intolerance .

Long story short, he had some nut allergies (which he barely ate anyway) but also had severe food intolerance reactions to both wheat and sugar, as well as a list of random foods. Let me tell you, in case you haven't been through a wheat-free/sugar-free diet, sugar and wheat are everywhere and in everything!

We took out all of the foods that weren't on the safe list our dietitian gave us, and within four days the tics started going away. Three weeks later, they were down to 5%. A month after that, they were gone completely. We have since reintroduced almost all of the foods except for his two severe foods, with no tics occurring. Everything he eats is organic. We also keep food coloring out. I am not suggesting that wheat and sugar are your problems, since everyone will have their own list of troublesome foods.

I want to cry when I think that I was sending my son to bed every night with a jam sandwich on wheat. But, I'm elated that we can move on, and that his future looks bright and clear.

I wanted to mention that we did try a multitude of diets in the past and none of them worked for us. Unless you know the exact foods that are a problem, there may be unknown multiple triggers. In that case, it is nearly impossible to sort out by removing just one item at a time. I know we went gluten-free for a while and there was no difference. Same with sugar. It wasn't until both these major trigger foods were out for a few days that we saw a difference.

Going organic was a key for us

JANICE: I want to share our success in eliminating 99.9% of tics with my daughter. I noticed her tics last year, when she had just turned nine. It started with shoulder-shrugging, throat-clearing, and blinking. It then moved on to hopping, jumping, and arm-jerking.

She would often drop things and had trouble reading because she would snap her head back sharply, and her hands jerked the pages until they tore. She would even swing her arms and accidentally hit people in stores. We did research, went to neurologists, tried supplements and a number of approaches. No change.

Then one day we went apple picking at an orchard. That day, and for almost two weeks afterwards, she had the worst tics ever. It got me thinking about pesticides. So we tried an organic diet.

After two weeks on the diet, there was a dramatic difference, but she still had tics. Then we realized: We should do organic 100%, down to the spices and the soy sauce and vitamins. Everything that she eats or drinks now is completely organic. And it works! Since we have tried this, she is essentially tic-free. When she has a tic it is mild, and usually we can pinpoint a food she ate, like a treat at a school birthday party. When this happens, we help her detox with an Epsom salt bath.

We have been on this diet for 6 months and I am confident that this is not a matter of spontaneous "waxing and waning." This diet is not easy. It's not cheap. It is completely inconvenient. It means that we have to home-cook every meal. We cannot eat out. Ever. We pack snacks, lunches, drinks, etc. Despite the inconvenience, I am beyond happy that we found the trigger.

We have to watch for hidden MSG

SURINDER: I realize that with Tourette's there can certainly be many causes, but in my son's case, who had tics for four years starting when he was three, MSG has to be avoided at all costs. I did food journals for months to try to figure out the pattern of why he was experiencing tics. All of a sudden it became very clear: so many of the products that gave him problems had MSG in them. Why is MSG such a problem? It is because it excites the nervous system.

A lot of people consider MSG to be simply a Chinese food issue. I can tell you that my 7-year-old son has never had Chinese food. The food industry uses MSG as a cheap food flavor enhancer. The biggest problem is that it is disguised under many different names other than MSG: Monosodium glutamate, monopotassium glutamate, glutamate, glutamic acid, hydrolyzed vegetable protein (HVP), gelatin, hydrolyzed plant protein (HPP), autolyzed plant protein, sodium caseinate, calcium caseinate, textured protein, yeast extract, yeast food or nutrient, and autolyzed yeast. All these are MSG under different names.

At one point my son started having some tics again and I could not figure out what was causing them. I had given him no MSG, or so I thought. Then I realized it was sodium caseinate (MSG) that is used in some whipped toppings. I had made a birthday cake and used the whipped topping from the store.

I learned from this that you even have to carefully check dairy products for sodium caseinate and calcium caseinate. I have also had to be a detective at my son's school for the school lunches. There was MSG in probably 70%+ of the lunches they serve. Also, for school parties you have to be aware of foods people might bring that could cause your child to react.

What I have had to do is read every food label like his life depends upon it, and also study all the names of MSG. I have had to research restaurants and which ones use MSG in their food. A great place to start researching these things is on migraine websites that focus on MSG. A lot of people get migraines from MSG, and I have found a great deal of information on these sites.

I can sum it all up with this simple sentence. When my son has his vitamins and minerals, and has no MSG, yellow 5, red 40, or high fructose corn syrup, he is virtually tic-free.

Corn was our son's problem

RONNIE: My son is going into sixth grade and has displayed motor tics since third grade, plus vocal tics. I noticed after he had some popcorn he started sniffing and clearing his throat nonstop. The allergy doctor tested him and found he was allergic to mold, trees, and cat, but a corn allergy did not show up. Still, I tried to have him avoid it and stopped serving whole corn. This year I started serving it again, and it triggered his Tourette symptoms intensely.

They were so bad, I don't know how he could read his school work. He would show no real signs while eating it, then hours later his symptoms would explode, with him humming, sniffing, sucking in air loudly (a whooping sound), and blinking. My son hasn't touched whole corn since, and he has been virtually symptom-free. Corn chips cause slight tics, but not enough to make him want to stop eating them.

ADHD medication trigger

My 7-year-old daughter was diagnosed with ADHD. She had trouble paying attention at school, and teachers thought she was missing out on instruction. She was also excitable. Our doctor suggested Strattera. We thought it would be safe because it is a nonstimulant drug, in contrast to Ritalin, which we had heard could cause tics to start up. Anyway, for us it was a big mistake. After a few days she developed head and arm shaking tics. They kept getting worse and I suspected the drug, even though I know it has helped others. We took her off of it, but it took months for the tics to stop.

After this, I read an article on *Latitudes.org* that had case reports from journals about tics being triggered from Strattera. I wish we had known. Now I see that Strattera has a black box warning for a risk of causing suicidal thoughts(!). Fortunately we did not have that problem, but it made me realize these drugs are not to be taken lightly by children, and some are very sensitive to them.

Reacting to chemicals, salicylates, and additives

VALERIE: My son was diagnosed with Tourette's shortly after turning seven. I remember when the tics started. It was after he had entered his first grade classroom right after the carpet had been cleaned, the room was painted, and new construction had been built to house a new central air conditioning unit without any ventilation. It was August and hot. After the unit was installed, the air had been turned on. All the construction dust, airborne contaminants from the carpet being cleaned, and outgassing from the paint circulated throughout the room. During this time he was also impulsive, moody, had night terrors, and was like the energizer bunny until he crashed at night.

After much research by me, my boy is now on a strict Feingold stage 1 diet (see *Feingold.org*). We are chemical-free at home and school. He is 13 and has been basically tic-free/symptom-free for 5 years, with the exception of when ant killer was spread on the playground beside him. This caused a tic that continued for about two months. Now he only at times has small shoulder twitching when playing sports or is extremely nervous, but that is all.

We learned that exposure to any synthetic fragrance or product like furniture polish, insecticides, pesticides, ant killer, air fresheners, and fragrant detergents/lotions/soaps could cause tics to resurface.

With foods, he is sensitive to salicylates (see page 168), sodium benzoate, and most preservatives, as well as artificial flavors, colors, and sweeteners.

Early on, we tried to explain to the neurologist that we were seeing symptom improvements. She immediately told us there is no research indicating environment causes the issue. We know with our son, it did.

I know what it's like to see your child struggle with symptoms of Tourette's. I now know the joy of seeing that same child live a normal life again. Be aware of what your child is exposed to, and you can help him or her live a healthy, more tic-free life. Thanks, *Latitudes*!

Chemical triggers

LAILA: My daughter started having tics at age 10. The tics began with just a small amount of finger-rolling when she spoke to us. Like an excited child, Dawn would hold her arms up and roll the thumb into the fingers. Then a mouth-grimacing movement developed. At age 11, she entered middle school, and the stress was tremendous. Vocal tics began.

Then, within a two-week span, we saw tics emerge at a frightening pace. Most tics were new ones we had never seen before. Previously, only one tic had appeared at a time, and now there were four or five at once. She would cry because her shoulder hurt from the relentless arm-jerking. Dawn complained of joint pain from moving her legs so much.

Soon my girl's head began moving, and she started blinking along with the other movements. Meanwhile, the vocal tics kept increasing. She made a sniffing sound and little animal-like sounds, like a guinea pig. We couldn't understand the rapid increase in tics; it was frightening.

At this point, my mother asked whether there might be a connection with our recent weight-loss diets. We were on a diet—both my daughter and I are overweight. At first I assured her there could not be a link, because one thing we did on this new diet was get rid of junk food. It seemed that was a good idea! But when my mother asked what we had replaced the junk food with, I realized something.

My family had all started on a health-conscious diet together, and Dawn lost ten pounds. We were keeping food diaries, watching "The Biggest Loser" on television, and exercising. The TV show had stressed the healthy addition of fat-free, low-calorie yogurt. At only 100 calories, it was a treat for Dawn in place of the sweets she used to enjoy. I also remembered that our daughter was now consuming no-calorie drinks made with tubes of powdered mix added to bottled water. I went to the cabinet and read the ingredients on these drink powders. There it was: aspartame (Nutrasweet/Equal). It was also in the so-called healthy yogurt. I called the pediatrician to report this discovery and was told I simply needed to accept her condition more fully. I kept pressing the issue, so finally the doctor conceded that if I was so concerned, I should pull them from the diet and see if it helped. I took care to remove all products that had any amount of aspartame under any of the several marketing names used at the time. This effort also eliminated many food dyes.

The effect was astounding. All tics decreased dramatically. Most stopped completely, and the verbal ones simply disappeared. I began to think about how my daughter has always been affected by chemicals on the outside of her body. She cannot use most shampoos or bath products, and has never been able to tolerate even bubble bath. If those chemicals affected her so much externally, didn't it make sense that chemicals could be causing her problems internally?

I began to watch for which foods did or did not affect her. After 30 days of no artificial sweeteners, I deliberately added aspartame to her diet, and immediately the tics came back, as bad as before. Then I removed it, and they went away as before.

I am no physician, but I'm not an idiot, either. I saw a vast change, like the flip of a switch. By keeping a food journal and making careful observations, I found other foods that trigger tics. Chocolate and sweets are among the top ones, and she seems to crave them. I've noticed that she has food-related mood swings. Previously we were told it was "just puberty" or premenstrual syndrome (PMS). Now I know better. Fatigue and stress also have an effect.

Aside from causing tics, troublesome foods can make her agitated. We now have an "avoid these foods" list. I actually believe this is a case of undiagnosed food allergy, or what I have dubbed "food toxicity." I believe my daughter was born with a sensitivity to many substances, some yet unknown to us. She is simply unable to handle the many unhealthy food additives in our food supply. I was so happy to find your *Latitudes.org* site, where so much information is available free of charge.

Dust as a key focus

I have a son who was normal until the age of 11. One day, he started heavy eye-blinking. Side mouth-twitching soon developed, then more serious tics, such as bending his head way to the side, and extreme shoulder shrugging. He later began repeating negative statements, over and over, and became high strung.

These symptoms continued for one year. At this point we decided medication would be better than the psychological damage he was experiencing. So, he began taking Clonidine. His tics diminished, but they were still enough for his peers to notice, and the drug side effects interrupted his social life.

In desperation, I began reading books on natural healing and allergies. My son is very allergic to dust mites. I covered his mattress and pillow, and removed dust from his bedroom. I began giving him some basic nutrients. His condition showed clear improvement with these changes, and he was able to reduce his Clonidine.

It has been a year, and he now has only occasional vocal tics (not in public), and 95% of the physical tics are gone. I feel that allergy plays a role in Tourette syndrome and that supplements can be helpful.

The environment, diet, and immune system

MARIA: My poor boy suffered through a lot. Tics started appearing at age three. By age seven he was doing horribly, with all-around multiple tics. He was walking on all fours because he was ticcing so much.

He was having a terrible time with allergies, and we were told he had asthma along with all his tics. Diet changes, including no dyes or preservatives, have helped my child. We went all-organic, and use healthy cleaning products. We put our son on a diet that reduced his allergies and sensitivities greatly.

We boosted his immune system with probiotics, and then in the long run he didn't get sick as often. My child never took an allergy medication, and his tics improved significantly.

I would be more than happy to stand in front of millions of people and say that my child's tics were helped by dietary changes, improving the immune system, and addressing environmental factors. If it wasn't for the *Latitudes.org* website to guide me, I fear what would have happened to my child.

Short notes from families

My child's tics started at age 6 when we began renovating our home. We had started in the basement with carpet, wallboards, and paint. Then we did the kitchen with new cabinets and counters. I noticed a lot of odor from both places. An allergist made the connection between the chemicals and tics, and told us how to minimize the exposure as best we could. The tics finally went away, but not my guilt. We are now all "natural" at home.

I wish I had known about an allergy connection to tics when I was a kid. I have significant allergies that I didn't realize were affecting my tics until I was in my 20s. I have a serious case of Tourette's and had never looked for triggers before then. About 10 years ago I realized that in addition to foods and allergens, electromagnetic fields were aggravating my tics as well.

I always knew that smoke made my son's tics worse, but I never thought about dust. I asked him to help me clean a very dusty area one day. By the time he was done clearing out months' worth of dust, his tics were out of control. Had I known, I would have done it myself. At least now I know he should wear a dust mask if he does clean.

Implementing information and suggestions provided on *Latitudes.org* **and** through your forums has equaled a tremendous amount of tic relief for our son, and given hope for our family. After researching, we tried alternative options which have mitigated motor tics 90-95%. Removal of all household chemicals, avoidance of milk, plus a mostly organic diet along with supplements, has worked wonders. Humbly we are not out of the woods but extremely hopeful.

I would say the main tic triggers are TV, artificial flavors and colors, MSG, corn syrup, and stress. We recently started the Feingold Diet and it seems to be helping tremendously when we stick to the brand names that the organization recommends.

We have a family history of Tourette's. My daughter reacted terribly to a used couch we brought into the home that had been freshly sprayed with Scotchguard® and smelled of scented plug-ins. We got rid of it immediately.

My child had a major exposure to mold at her elementary school that resulted in muscle spasms and made her prone to chronic infections that have been difficult to treat. I've had to home-school her. Her spasms are much better when away from the school.

My daughters and I are able to control our tics simply by eliminating artificial colors, flavors, and the preservatives BHA, BHT, and TBHQ. I suggest you make any dietary changes gradually, not doing too many at once. Read labels, and if you see anything like Red #40 or Yellow #5, then find an organic or all-natural substitute. Remember that most pickles list Yellow #5 as an ingredient! Keep a food diary and record everything your child eats and drinks, along with noting symptoms. A diary/log can be a good tool for identifying triggers or patterns to the symptoms.

Eliminating certain foods has made a big difference for my son's tics. Foods he needs to avoid based upon testing done over a year ago: cane sugar, milk and milk products from any animal, rice and rice products, corn and corn products, grains and any product that contains gluten. Also, soy products and mushrooms. The foods that he showed sensitivity to during testing did prove to be triggers for tics. As a result of avoiding them, his sleep has also improved, he has a lot less stomach pains, and behavior is consistent (which is now a sweet temperament).

I am from China and the mother of a seventeen-year-old boy who has been afflicted with Tourette syndrome for some years. Over the years of struggle, I noticed some things triggered his tics more than others, for sure. The biggest offender is allergic reaction caused by air pollution, and then colds—especially when his nose is affected.

My boy has Tourette's and tested negative for PANDAS (see pages 114-116) seven years ago. He is able to get his omega-3 from flaxseed oil and from his diet, but he cannot take any form of fish oil, as it triggers tics for him, even though he can eat fish with no problem. I know this has also been reported by others who have Tourette's, although some can take fish oil with no problem.

When my son is ill he tics more, and then these triggers surface for him: television, stress(!), excitement, doing homework, and, I believe, artificial food coloring. When he is healthy, he can tolerate these things without a problem. His brother has PANDAS, and strep infections set off this son's tics. He then gets red ears, increased vocal throat tics, and has a short temper. These symptoms seem to happen after orange juice, tomatoes, or grape juice, all foods in the salicylates category (see page 168 for more on salicylates).

I always dread allergy season, not just because of the annoying symptoms of itchy eyes, cough, and runny nose, but because it makes my tics worse. It is a cycle that repeats every year. I've also noticed that my tics are better or worse depending on what part of the country I live in.

While we were on the GAPS diet, my child's tics became undetectable. (GAPS stands for gut and psychology syndrome.) The improvement was so gradual that one day I realized that I couldn't remember the last time I had noticed a tic. We are now on a low carb, gluten-free, soy-free diet. This past year, as long as he is off soy, the tics and OCD are unnoticeable to me. It has been a lot of work to change the way we eat, but so worth it. Soy was definitely not on our radar as a tic trigger at first; it is worth eliminating soy as a trial to see if it helps.

For my son, food additives were causing him to tic, with artificial colors being at the top of the list, artificial flavors next, and a host of others following suit (like preservatives, synthetic vitamins, etc.). All the neurologists and psychiatrists we saw told me that we were imagining this. The tics were so severe (head jerking, hand and arm tics, and vocal tics) that he was willing to go on a very "pure" diet. Over time, the tics have greatly diminished. It used to be that one tiny bit of a chemical additive would cause a problem that took days to eradicate. Now it takes larger amounts to cause the tics, and they go away quickly upon stopping the offending item.

We have seen a definite decrease in a chronic vocal tic disorder by greatly reducing TV time and eliminating video games for our child. When he recently played video games on my iPad, his tics escalated within an hour of playing, and persisted at an increased level for days. It seems it doesn't matter what system is used for the video games (iPad, computer, console, etc.), they can all result in tic escalation for him.

My son's tic, which he had for 3 years before the start of a cascade of other neurological symptoms, went away after cutting out wheat. No tests recommended by his doctor showed any problems, from blood work, to a CT scan, to an EEG. It sickens me that diet is not the first treatment considered for neurological, psychiatric, and behavioral conditions.

My 10-year-old child has had significant tics since age 2. I have always wanted to try to lessen tics through nonpharmacologic means. About eight months ago, we took away all artificial colors and flavors, and took away gluten, dairy, and corn. I have been amazed at the improvement. Not only have the tics almost vanished, but migraines, hyperactivity, agitation, and overall mood improved. I tried to reintroduce popcorn (since we all LOVE popcorn) and even though it was organic, which is non-GMO, it did not go well. Even he felt the difference. It is not an easy diet to follow, but it's been SO worth it!

I read the ACN book *Natural Treatments for Tics & Tourette's* **and have kept** a food diary for my daughter. This has been a huge help. Triggers, in addition to foods, are excitement or stress, strong smells, and pollens.

I was diagnosed with Tourette syndrome at age 38 (I am now 64). I have found that diet does indeed have an impact on the severity of my tics. Petroleum products like gas, diesel, oil-based paints and stains, etc., also bother me. Four years ago I found out about light sensitivity, often known as Irlen Syndrome. I have been wearing Irlen filters (lenses) for 3 1/2 years and the reduction of my tics has been astounding. (For more information: *Irlen.com*)

My son, now 15, has had OCD and Tourette's since he was five. He has also always suffered from sinus issues, having numerous rounds of antibiotics when he was four. He does not have any "true allergies" but does react to many things in the environment, including VOCs (volatile organic compounds that are often toxic, as in paints), stress, and certain foods.

We have had a huge success following the Specific Carbohydrate Diet (SCD) for the past 15 months. If you decide to follow the SCD, give it one month. This was all I asked of my son. The first two weeks were absolutely horrible and it all got much worse, but by the end of the month, he had seen enough improvement that he wanted to continue (and still does).

I am an adult with tics and have to avoid most department stores. The lighting is often much too bright, and it is almost impossible to avoid the smells from the cosmetics department; this aggravates me. Smaller stores, like gift stores, can be really bad also, with all their scented candles and potpourri. I'm grateful for online shopping! I also find that plug-ins in public bathrooms and even in friends' homes are a tic trigger for me.

I found that exposure to standard insect repellent could make my son's facial and neck tics worse. It was repeatedly sprayed on him at school because the staff thought they had to protect students when they went out to play at recess. He would come home from school with a major increase in tics. It took some detective work before I figured it out and gave the school a safer product to use.

My daughter's tics are definitely helped, though not cured, through diet. As well as having nothing artificial, we did an elimination diet and found she reacted strongly to wheat, eggs, dairy, and corn. Corn, by the way, seems to be in everything in America! Eliminating these foods that were bothering her, and eating "super clean," has made her tics invisible to most people. I would really recommend an elimination diet to see if there are things that are aggravating your tics.

Tics can be triggered by preservatives, and I have found one of the worst is calcium disodium EDTA. This preservative is used in almost all margarine and mayonnaise. For myself, one instance of consumption can last more than three weeks. As a rule, I generally do not eat anything containing it. I need to avoid many restaurants, like a popular chicken chain that used EDTA in all its sauces and mayonnaise. It seems many places use certain mayo and margarines without being aware of the EDTA. It is also used in some iced teas, energy drinks, and canned products (read all the labels!). I find that dye-free Benadryl capsules help me when I am having a reaction.

Our son seemed healthy, but when he was six years old he developed some mild tics. By the fourth grade, something had gone terribly wrong. He disrupt-ed his gifted classes with ear-splitting shrieks. He made noises, kicked desks, and waved his arms. For six weeks the tics were so bad that he couldn't even hold a pencil. He was depressed and wished he were dead. And all this was while he was on medication. He saw two allergists. He was found with testing to have an allergic reaction to several foods, and each caused different tic symptoms. Apple and chocolate brought on some of the worst tics. My son was also hypersensitive to certain dusts, molds, pollens, and chemicals. With avoidance and allergy treatment, he now leads a normal life. *(From Ginger Wakem, whose pioneering efforts grew into ACN:* Latitudes.org)

Our 15-year old son has had Tourette's since he was 9. He now avoids milk due to a high whey sensitivity, and also wheat products. He has a very dramatic reaction to synthetic folate (labeled specifically "Folic Acid"), which is in every form of commercially sold bread and pasta product in the U.S. This additive is mandated by the FDA to prevent spina bifida. We eliminated items with this ingredient and saw marked improvement. Weeks later, he accidentally ingested it in some breaded chicken. He experienced a four-day severe bout of tics; the connection was very obvious. We have learned he is unable to tolerate this type of folate.

The biggest mistake of our life was giving our son Abilify for his serious tics. This drug is an antipsychotic that is sometimes used for Tourette syndrome. He did not have any signs of psychosis or depression but the doctor prescribed it anyway. (This was years ago, before we knew anything about allergic reactions causing tics, or food triggers—although we had seen that sugar made his tics very severe.) Anyway, his reaction to Abilify was frightening and the nightmare has not stopped. Not only did it not help his tics, but he developed additional tics and movements along with extreme anxiety and OCD. If you look up the side-effects to this drug you can see what it can trigger. Sadly, these seem to be permanent effects and nothing we have been able to do has helped him recover from this drug. He is truly disabled from it.

While remodeling our home, we pulled up an old carpet (moldy and dusty). Our nine-year-old son suddenly developed such severe tics that we had to take him to the hospital emergency room. We have since learned a great deal about his allergies. In our case, there has been a definite benefit from an environmental approach.

Our child was dealing with a candida overgrowth problem, assessed with a urine test. The doctor explained how a "leaky gut" can affect the nervous system. He treated the problem with an antifungal prescription medication, and we had to reduce all sugars. I used to think drinking fruit juice was good, then learned how much sugar is in it, so we started diluting it, just using a little for flavoring. Avoiding the candida triggers has made a major improvement in his tics.

Eliminating allergens has helped with our son's tics. We removed our carpets, got rid of a down comforter, and have done battle with bathroom mold. Eliminating artificial colors and flavors, dairy, and corn syrup as best as we could, helped with behavior. After these changes, his lip-licking tics (the most obvious) which for the past six years have tended to be worse in the fall until the first frost, were not as pronounced this past fall.

A blood pressure medication prescribed to control the tics seemed to make my son weepy and aggressive. A couple of years ago, after reading Daniel G. Amen's book *Healing ADHD*, I agreed to a trial of Prozac. The results of Prozac on behavior have been pretty dramatic. I am convinced there's some sort of allergy link to his tics. We have found our answer by combining traditional drug therapy with non-conventional approaches.

We changed our family diet so there is no wheat, dairy, food coloring, or processed foods, and no refined sugar. Sound familiar? The doctor also put our son on a number of supplements, some of which are natural anti-inflammatory agents and calm his nervous system.

Within weeks the results were mind-blowing. Five to six simultaneous simple and complex motor and phonic tics were reduced to one motor tic. A year later I keep waiting for the other shoe to drop at peak periods, like school starting or holidays. But there is still only one tic, sometimes none.

I think we could probably eradicate tics altogether if we were more diligent, but we follow an 80/20 rule with the restrictions. It's a good balance for us; his only tic is not noticeable to him or others and we are not robbing him and his brothers of every joy in life at things like birthday parties and eating out.

A *note from the author*: I have published the closing letter below a number of times. It was first received by the Tourette Syndrome Association in the 1990s. Eleanor Pearl, one of the original founders of that organization, sent it to me because she wanted to be sure that it would be shared. I include it here to honor both Mrs. Pearl's request, although she has since passed away, as well as the writer's heartfelt wish.

I suffered from the embarrassment of Tourette's all my life. I'm 42 and a medical technician. 15 years ago I changed my eating habits; I drastically reduced refined foods/red meat and ate more raw fruits and veggies. I started nutritional supplements. But it wasn't until I stopped consuming corn syrup, especially high fructose corn syrup, that my symptoms almost entirely subsided. Do not think this is "all in my head." I am well aware of the placebo effect and can assure you that this was not the case. Please do not let this letter end up in a wastebasket. I feel strongly others could be helped.

In closing: A matter of choice

Latitudes was selected as the name for our organization's newsletter and website because one meaning of the term "latitude" is *freedom of action or choice.*

The decision to make an effort to identify and avoid environmental and dietary triggers is a matter of personal choice. As some of the writers explain in their testimonials, the process of finding triggers and then making adjustments to avoid them is not always easy, and the path not always clear.

As with many areas of health, some people are willing to make lifestyle changes in the hope that new efforts will be helpful. Others are not willing, or are unable to do so, for any number of understandable reasons.

ACN simply promotes the concept of choice, and people cannot choose if they do not know their options.

There is no need to "protect" the tic community from these types of reports. In fact, the more who know of these potential connections, the greater the chances of self-discovery and the greater the opportunity for advancement in the global understanding of tics.

Additional trigger experiences are included in *Natural Treatments for Tics & Tourette's: A Patient and Family Guide,* as well as on our website and forums at *www.Latitudes.org.* ACN continues to receive trigger reports such as those in this chapter.

For these accounts the writers implemented change, monitored for a response, and then took the time to share their findings with us. As time goes on, some may need to tweak their observations. They may have setbacks and need to reassess their next steps. But each knows that in his or her case, there are at least some answers to the "mystery" of tics, and with this knowledge they are in a better position to move forward in reducing symptoms.

With increased education on the topic of triggers, the tic community will feel more empowered to look for clues to symptoms. Medical professionals will also be in a better position to help patients deal with tics, and new discoveries are sure to be made.

What is clear, based on the current absence of research efforts in this area (see the next chapter), is that those who insist on the publication of definitive studies before considering a personal search for tic triggers will be in for a very long wait. That decision, of course, is also a matter of choice.

Notes

Tourette Syndrome

Section Three

Where is the research?

Types of tic triggers

How can there be so many triggers?

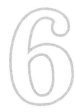

Where is the research?

At times I have been asked why ACN (*Latitudes.org*) shares personal reports and survey results rather than focusing on scientific journals as the primary source of information on tic triggers. The reason for this is simple. Only minimal research on this topic has been published.

I suggest that perhaps the greatest "mystery" surrounding tic disorders is that such little creative thought has been given to discovering *why* symptoms wax and wane. It is a major disservice to those affected that tic triggers have been largely ignored by the scientific community. But, the lack of research is definitely not our organization's fault. We have repeatedly encouraged studies in this area, to little avail.

It is important for the reader to understand how utterly disengaged and disinterested the medical community and key advocacy groups appear to be related to issues of diet, allergy, toxins, and other potential daily influences on tics. While these subjects do not tend to garner the same level of research funding as pharmaceuticals do, studies on triggers and related topics have moved forward for many other medical conditions.

The Tourette Association of America announced in June 2017 that they have awarded a total of 21 million dollars for studies on genetics. Unfortunately, progress in genetic studies has been slow. Meanwhile, they have not funded research on the topics highlighted in this book. The one exception is one inconclusive study on essential fatty acids for Tourette's.

Comparison charts on research interest

Graphs in this chapter reflect research interests for a range of relevant issues related to Tourette's. While the incidence for conditions specified in the charts varies, nevertheless the data reveal a serious lack of leadership in this field.

As previously mentioned, it is widely accepted that risk factors for Tourette's are not solely genetic, but as much as 40% environmental, making this an obvious target for research. And, up to 90% of patients with Tourette's have additional co-morbid conditions, most commonly ADHD and OCD. Given this, it would be logical to pursue similar areas of research for Tourette's as, for example, for ADHD. ADHD research is highlighted in these charts. Has the field of Tourette syndrome kept pace? Judge for yourself. Note that ADHD studies have had a particular focus on environmental and dietary factors.

Comparisons with migraine research

In addition to ADHD, migraine also has an association with Tourette's. As indicated on page 23, there is a fourfold increase in incidence of headache and migraine among children and adolescents with Tourette's. We should be exploring some of the same research areas for tics as occur for migraine. You can compare the charts to see how the field of Tourette's measures up.

The graphs are based on the number of research articles produced by a September 2017 search on *PubMed.gov* for Tourette syndrome, as well as for the other conditions indicated. **Note:** *PubMed.gov* provides abstracts and at times the full text of research articles. The number of studies obtained from a PubMed search is typically greater than the total that actually focus on a given topic. This is because other loosely related articles are often included in search results. With this in mind, the graphs presented are to be used only for general comparison purposes to reflect the scientific "interest" in the topics.

There is not a direct one-to-one comparison for each element of these charts. For example, there is currently a greater incidence of autism than Tourette's. Conversely, more people have a diagnosis of Tourette syndrome than have the movement disorder Parkinson's disease. Yet, Parkinson's research has seen a much greater focus on diverse factors including allergy, diet, the environment, pesticides, pollution, and triggers than Tourette syndrome research has.

Clearly, studies on Tourette's for the topics highlighted in these charts are negligible. The tic community should ask: What excuse could there be for this?

Keep in mind: Here is where things stand after 45 years of advocacy for tic disorders

- Gene research "breakthroughs" in Tourette syndrome currently apply to a very small percentage in the Tourette community and are at the preliminary stage of discovery. The findings do not yet directly impact patients and families as far as prevention and treatment of symptoms.

- Subgroups for tic disorders that could help identify different causes and best treatment approaches have not been clearly defined.

- Effective medications without unwanted side effects are not currently available.

- 40% of Tourette's is understood to be "environmental," but this issue has barely been studied for tic disorders. While recent research has started to explore immune connections, helpful guidelines and recommendations have not been provided to the public with regard to the role of the environment and tics.

Tourette syndrome is now considered a common condition, with prevalence estimates being as high as 1 in 100 (See pages 9-10).

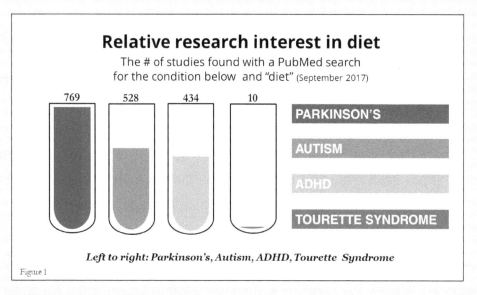

Relative research interest in diet

The # of studies found with a PubMed search
for the condition below and "diet" (September 2017)

769 528 434 10

PARKINSON'S

AUTISM

ADHD

TOURETTE SYNDROME

Left to right: Parkinson's, Autism, ADHD, Tourette Syndrome

Figure 1

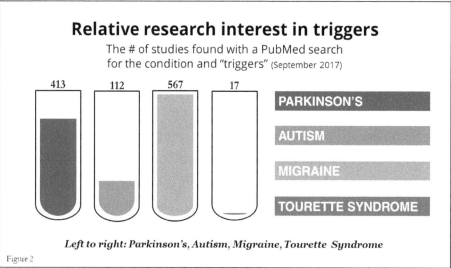

Relative research interest in triggers

The # of studies found with a PubMed search
for the condition and "triggers" (September 2017)

413 112 567 17

PARKINSON'S

AUTISM

MIGRAINE

TOURETTE SYNDROME

Left to right: Parkinson's, Autism, Migraine, Tourette Syndrome

Figure 2

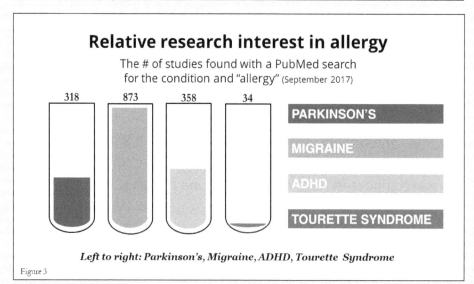

Relative research interest in allergy

The # of studies found with a PubMed search
for the condition and "allergy" (September 2017)

318 873 358 34

PARKINSON'S

MIGRAINE

ADHD

TOURETTE SYNDROME

Left to right: Parkinson's, Migraine, ADHD, Tourette Syndrome

Figure 3

The research interest for environmental impacts on Tourette syndrome lags far behind other conditions, even though it accounts for at least 40% of the developmental risk. (See page 1).

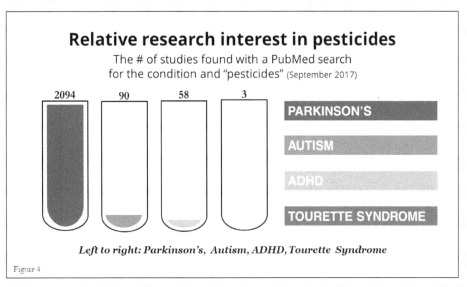

Relative research interest in pesticides

The # of studies found with a PubMed search
for the condition and "pesticides" (September 2017)

2094   90   58   3

PARKINSON'S

AUTISM

ADHD

TOURETTE SYNDROME

Left to right: Parkinson's, Autism, ADHD, Tourette Syndrome

Figure 4

Relative research interest in environment

The # of studies found with a PubMed search
for the condition and "environment" (September 2017)

1944   1971   1468   111

PARKINSON'S

AUTISM

ADHD

TOURETTE SYNDROME

Left to right: Parkinson's, Autism, ADHD, Tourette Syndrome

Figure 5

Relative research interest in pollution

The # of studies found with a PubMed search
for the condition below and "pollution" (September 2017)

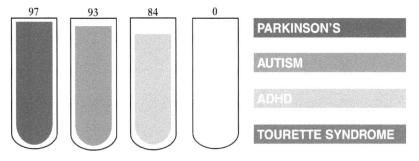

97   93   84   0

PARKINSON'S

AUTISM

ADHD

TOURETTE SYNDROME

Left to right: Parkinson's, Autism, ADHD, Tourette Syndrome

Figure 6

Moving forward

The study of tics and Tourette syndrome needs to move in new directions if we are to discover the underlying causes of tics and provide more effective approaches to prevention and treatment.

When it became clear that the incidence of autism was rising at an alarming rate, media coverage was widespread and studies on the influence of the environment in the disorder began in earnest. We are looking at a similar rapid rise in the prevalence of tics and Tourette syndrome. Where is the media coverage on this increase? Where is the research? Where is the leadership?

Types of tic triggers

Our organization's online survey (2003) documenting triggers for tics was completed by 1,789 participants. It was the first of its kind and has yet to be replicated. Since publishing the results in *Natural Treatments for Tics & Tourette's: A Patient and Family Guide*, we have collected additional trigger reports through our *Latitudes.org* forums and online correspondence, and at conferences. This feedback has been incorporated into the trigger lists provided here.

Allergic, dietary and environmental tic triggers are not yet addressed in conventional medical literature. As a result, one could assume that many respondents would not have been actively looking for a cause-and-effect relationship for tic symptoms when they completed our survey. This is in contrast to studies in which a participant is instructed to keep a log for a number of weeks to determine triggers, and then report on any noted associations.

With this in mind, it is likely that some survey respondents were experiencing triggers that they were completely unaware of. As such, the lists provided in this chapter may omit some potential triggers. At the other end of the spectrum, there is always the possibility that someone assumed there was a connection with a given influence at the time they completed the survey, but then further observations changed their impressions.

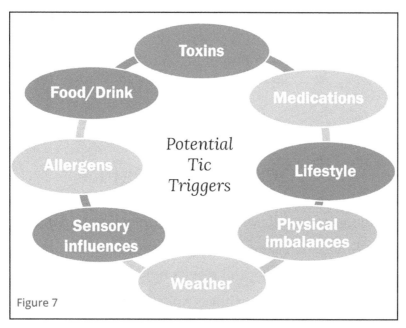

Figure 7

Trigger categories

Are the trigger lists offered here complete and definitive? No. Do they confirm that triggers exist for tic symptoms just as they do for many other medical conditions? Yes, absolutely.

The diagnostic label "Tourette syndrome" is an umbrella term that no doubt covers a number of subsets that are yet to be identified. Future research may show that one subset of people with tics is more prone to certain types of triggers than another subset, but that has not yet been determined.

Multiple types or categories of triggers can impact someone, as well as can multiple items within a given category. Eight types of triggers are shown in the chart above and are included in our breakdown of trigger types on the following pages, with toxins and allergens grouped together.

Some trigger categories may overlap; there are items that could fall under more than one type. Although the groupings are somewhat arbitrary, we hope these categories are helpful.

Lifestyle triggers for tics

- Anxiety
- Car: new (outgassing toxins)
- Car or bus rides
- Cell phone use
- Computer/tablet use
- Disrupted sleep
- Doing nothing (boredom)
- Electromagnetic fields
- Electronic exposures
- Emotional states
- Excitement
- Fatigue
- Homes: newly built, moldy, remodeled, with allergens
- Hunger/hypoglycemia
- Lack of regular meals
- Motion sickness
- Overstimulation
- Pollution exposure
- Reading
- Showers with treated water
- Smoking and secondhand smoke; lingering smoke odors
- Stress: mental and emotional
- Television viewing
- Video gaming (*See also visual stimulation in Sensory Triggers, below*)

Sensory triggers for tics

- Eating: specific food textures, swallowing
- Fragrances
- Listening to talk about tics
- Listening to certain music (i.e., fast techno beat)
- Odors of chemicals or foods (*see also Toxic and Allergic Triggers page 91*)
- Seeing other people tic
- Sounds and noise
- Sweating
- Tastes, certain flavors
- Temperature, especially heat; a big change between indoor and outdoor temperatures
- Touch: clothing and other items on skin; human touch
- Visual stimulation (photo sensitivity), television and monitors, tablet screens and cell phones, flickering lights, stadium night lights, headlights, watching movies in a theater, video games

Food and beverage triggers for tics

- Alcohol
- Apples
- Artificial colors
- Artificial flavors
- Avocados
- Bananas
- Beer
- Caffeine
- Cane sugar
- Cheeses, especially aged
- Chicken
- Chocolate
- Cinnamon
- Citrus fruits
- Corn
- Dairy products
- Eggs
- Fermented and pickled foods; sauerkraut
- Fish, smoked
- Gluten-containing foods
- High-fructose corn syrup
- Meats, processed
- Monosodium glutamate (see pages 59-60, 166)
- Nitrates/nitrites
- Nutrasweet/aspartame
- Non-organic foods
- Peanuts/peanut butter
- Preservatives BHT, BHA, AND TBHQ, sodium nitrate
- Salicylates (see page 168)
- Sesame
- Smoked meats
- Sodas: sugary, artificially sweetened or flavored, caffeinated
- Soy
- Spices
- Strawberries
- Sweets, in general
- Tomato
- Tyramine-containing foods
- Vinegars
- Wheat
- Wine
- Yeast-containing foods

Toxic and allergic triggers for tics

- Aftershave, cologne
- Air fresheners: plug-in type, aerosol, car deodorizers and other conventional forms
- Air quality: poor, smog
- Animal dander: pets like cat, dog, rabbit, hamster
- Candles: chemically-scented, petroleum-based
- Carpet: new or when cleaning, removal of old (moldy/dusty)
- Chlorine and bleach
- Cleaning products
- Deodorants
- Dust
- Exhaust; diesel and other gasoline fumes
- Fabric softener
- Facial cleansers
- Formaldehyde
- Hair products, hair sprays
- Herbicides
- Incense
- Insect bites
- Kerosene fumes
- Furniture: new, treated fabric
- Laundry detergent: scented
- Molds
- Paint and paint thinners
- Perfumes
- Pesticides; insect repellent
- Pine trees
- Pollens: trees, ragweed, etc.
- Remodeling: glues, caulking, varnishes, paints, pressed board cabinets, flooring, etc.
- Sunscreen

See also Medications, page 92

Weather-related triggers for tics

- Allergy seasons
- Barometric pressure changes
- Bright sunlight
- Changes in humidity
- Changes in temperature
- Heat
- Rain
- Seasonal changes

Physical-related triggers for tics

- Candida overgrowth
- Dental: getting spacers, braces, sealants, fillings; losing teeth
- Fatigue
- Fever
- Hormonal changes
- Infections: viral, bacterial, parasitic; Lyme, strep, other
- Jaw misalignment
- Low blood sugar
- Muscle pain and fatigue from ticcing
- Structural misalignments, in general

Medications that might trigger tics

- Allergy medications
- Antidepressants
- Antihistamines
- Antipsychotics
- Aspirin
- Asthma medications
- Cold medicines; decongestants
- Heartburn meds: (Prevacid)
- Laxatives
- Lice treatment
- Medicated shampoos
- Stimulant medications
- Vaccines: next column

On vaccines

Reports of vaccines as tic triggers have been informally self-reported to ACN, including the tetanus, Flumist, Hepatitis B, and MMR.

Research has implicated vaccines containing the preservative thimerosal as a cause of tics.[30-33]

In addition, a key 2017 study showed a temporal association between vaccines and the onset of some pediatric-onset neuropsychiatric disorders, including anorexia nervosa, OCD, anxiety disorders, and tic disorders.[34]

Personal thresholds for reactions to triggers can fluctuate based on a number of health and emotional/mental factors. Also, keep in mind that food intolerances or sensitivities may shift and improve or worsen over time.

An individual does not always react to the same trigger with the same severity during each trigger episode. The degree of either resistance or susceptibility to a trigger varies with the strength of the immune system and other factors which can change. It is best to keep a log and monitor reactions to exposures over time to see an overall pattern.

Once you determine something is a trigger, the golden rule is "avoidance, avoidance, avoidance." This, of course, is in addition to efforts taken to reduce overall sensitivity through integrative medical interventions.

Increases in tics due to medications

Recent journal articles suggest that stimulant medications used to treat ADHD, such as Ritalin, do not, in fact, cause or worsen tic disorders. For many years, these drugs have been suspected of having this negative effect. The argument now being made is that tics frequently occur along with ADHD, with or without stimulant medication. However, not all families would agree with this new viewpoint, based on their personal experience of observing that tics developed or worsened after the use of stimulant or other drugs for ADHD began.

Meanwhile, limited case reports of medications triggering tics point a finger at the drugs Zoloft and Lexapro, in select cases. Families should also be aware that in addition to single drugs causing tics in susceptible individuals, a combination of medications can have a synergistic effect and result in side effects not usually experienced when a drug is taken in isolation. If you believe a medication is connected to an increase in tics, be sure to tell your prescribing physician.

Notes

How can there be so many triggers?

I believe readers will appreciate the following personal account. The writer had initially reacted negatively when he learned of the large number of possible triggers for tics. His report "Rethinking Triggers for Tourette Syndrome" is published on *Latitudes.org* in our Families Speak Out section for Tourette's.

> **BLAKE:** I had tics as a kid, but they were never diagnosed at the time. My mother simply called them nervous habits, which she and her mother also had. But mine were complex tics, mostly involving my eyes and hands, and some were vocal. I later received a diagnosis of Tourette syndrome.
>
> I have tried 14 psychiatric drugs. Some of these medications actually made the symptoms worse. I've also tried acupuncture and homeopathy, but they only seemed to help me short-term.
>
> I reached a point in my thirties wherein, even with different medications, my tics were very bad for five years straight. They were tormenting me, and I really needed help. I finally found the book *Natural Treatments for Tics & Tourette's* by Sheila Rogers DeMare. But, I made the "mistake" of starting my reading with the chapter on triggers!
>
> For those who haven't seen it, Sheila's organization did a large survey and published a list of many different things that people reported could trigger their tics. There were so many possibilities, because people are so different —from scented products to food additives to dust to chlorine. I immediately felt discouraged.

I didn't know where to start in looking at the triggers—I was so overwhelmed. So, I turned to the *ACN Latitudes* forums to vent. I remember griping that I thought it was absurd that there were so many trigger options to consider. Someone responded that what she thought was absurd was that doctors prescribe drugs for tics that can have terrible side effects, plus the drugs never got to the actual cause of the tics.

She had a point. Many people helped me out, and the support I received on the forum allowed me to forge ahead and finish reading the book. I read: "In some people a single trigger can aggravate or set off tics, while for others, several triggers may be present at the same time. Naturally, the level and duration of exposure to a trigger also makes a difference."

What a turnaround. By the time I finished *Natural Treatments for Tics & Tourette's* I was encouraged. It was incredible. I could relate to so much of what was written. My favorite section was the testimonials. It seemed that many families had reduced their tics by eliminating certain foods—whatever the person was most sensitive to. Wheat and dairy were often mentioned. I had started the blood-type diet (Eat Right 4 Your Type) for health reasons just a few months before, and I noticed my tics had been reduced a little.

I now looked at my diet even more closely. I eliminated wheat, dairy, corn, and potatoes, and tried to avoid caffeine.

I was thrilled to find that my tics subsided. I knew I was on the right path, and soon I was able to enjoy being tic-free. It has now been three years and I'm still tic-free as long as I eat "clean." Too much stress, caffeine, and toxic foods will cause a flare. I'm doing so much better. I have come to realize that people will do just about anything to feel "well" except change what they eat. In my opinion, it is truly the most difficult thing to change about a person. But it can also be so important.

I would encourage each person with a tic disorder to have an open mind. Look into possible triggers. It is worth the effort to learn what could be aggravating your tics.

Comment on the previous account: It is understandable to feel overwhelmed at the thought of a trigger search. As encouraging as it is to know that triggers might be increasing the tic response, and that their elimination could potentially improve or eliminate symptoms, the needed detective work can seem daunting. Regardless of whether you focus initially on diet, allergy, or chemical exposures, some degree of effort and attention will be required.

Many parents and patients have worked wonders reducing tics by identifying triggers on their own. Another option is to seek professional help from an allergist, environmental physician, or integrative practitioner. (See *www. Latitudes.org/trigger-resources* for links with referral information.) Receiving peer support on our *Latitudes.org* forums can also be helpful.

Why are people so allergic these days?

Instead of asking why there are so many possible triggers listed in Chapter 7, perhaps we should be asking, "Why are so many people allergic these days?"

It is estimated that worldwide, as many as one in three now experience allergies at some point during their life. Allergy is caused when the body's immune system reacts to a normally harmless substance. The body identifies it as a threat, and an exaggerated response to it is produced. The nervous system has always had the potential to be negatively affected by a variety of agents as diverse as, for example, gasoline odors, corn, molds, and dog dander. Yet there are many more complaints of allergy and environmentally-based illnesses now than there were decades ago. Correspondingly, we know that the incidence of tic disorders has increased dramatically.

Researchers have suggested a number of factors that might be responsible for the increase in allergy. There is no consensus on the cause(s). Theories include the "hygiene hypothesis," which proposes that living conditions are now too clean, and as a result, children are not exposed to enough germs or allergens to stimulate the body's positive immune responses. Other explanations being explored include, in part, increased use of antibiotics, the wide use of acetaminophen (Tylenol), vitamin D deficiencies, and varying environmental exposures during fetal development and early childhood, including electromagnetic radiation. The role of vaccines in the dramatic increase in immune and autoimmune disorders remains controversial and is receiving increased scrutiny.

A complex relationship among genetic, immunological, environmental, emotional, and infectious factors can impact the delicate nervous system.

Complaints of responses to odors and other chemicals

Research by Dr. Anne Steinemann (March 2017) indicated that 33% of Australians complain of health problems such as migraine and asthma attacks when exposed to fragranced products. These products include items such as air fresheners and deodorizers, personal care products, cleaning supplies, laundry products, household products, and others with "fragrance" added. A typical fragrance, she said, is usually a mixture of several dozen to several hundred chemicals. Even green or so-called organic products can emit hazardous pollutants if they contain fragrances. While touted to improve air quality, in fact they do the opposite. Widespread support for fragrance-free environments was reported.[35]

An increasing number of studies are being devoted to odors and their effects on the nervous system. In studies of patients with migraine, 70% to 90% had a migraine triggered by chemical odors. The worst offenders were perfumes, cleaning products, cigarette smoke, paints, gasoline, and motor vehicle exhaust.[36,37] Please note that these same types of odors were reported as tic triggers in our lists in Chapter 7.

The TILT theory: Do not dismiss low levels of exposures

Low levels of exposures can be surprisingly problematic. When thinking of triggers, there is a tendency to assume that only major, or what appear to be "significant," amounts of something can cause a reaction. Yet, Dr. Claudia Miller, co-author of the groundbreaking book *Low Levels, High Stakes*,[38] asserts that many people have developed a hypersensitivity to even low levels of environmental and allergic exposures. These levels can be so low that one might not suspect they could cause a reaction—so low in fact, that others may not believe (or may even ridicule) complaints or reports of a reaction.

Dr. Miller proposes that exposure to chemicals has created this widespread hypersensitivity. The exposure could either be from a major single event, or from ongoing chronic exposure to one or more lower levels of chemicals. "Today," she says, "we are witnessing a medical anomaly—a unique pattern of illness involving chemically-exposed groups, in more than a dozen countries, who subsequently report multi-system symptoms and new-onset chemical, food, and drug intolerances."

Dr. Miller refers to this condition as Toxicant-Induced Loss of Tolerance (TILT). She suggests that first there is a breakdown in prior tolerance due to either an acute or chronic exposure to chemicals like pesticides, solvents, or indoor air contaminants. This is followed by a triggering of symptoms when exposed to small quantities of factors that previously were tolerated. These items could be, for example, traffic exhaust, fragrances, foods, drugs, and food/drug combinations. Dr. Miller indicates that multiple neurotransmitter pathways may be involved in this response.[39]

I first read about Dr. Miller in Peter Radetsky's excellent book, *Allergic to the Twentieth Century*.[40] Published 20 years ago, Radetsky described multiple chemical sensitivity, Gulf War syndrome, sick building syndrome, and the plight of nearly 40 million Americans reported to react to common chemicals.

At the time of Radetsky's writing, mainstream medicine was hell-bent on disproving the claims of those who insisted chemical exposures were negatively affecting them, as well as discrediting the doctors who treated them. This hot topic included complaints by veterans from the 1991 Persian Gulf War. It has taken many years for hundreds of thousands of vets to receive disability benefits and the recognition that the illnesses they described were not simply psychological. The number of people reacting with physical symptoms to chemicals has increased, yet the controversy remains.

The special challenges of electronic screens

My book, *Natural Treatments for Tics & Tourette's: A Patient and Family Guide* includes reports from parents who observed that their child ticced more when watching TV and/or playing video games. Dr. Victoria Dunckley, an integrative child and adult psychiatrist in Los Angeles, concurs.

Based on her research and clinical work, Dr. Dunckley indicates that exposure to screens such as those from mobile devices, computers, and video games, can increase tics. Her book, *Reset Your Child's Brain*[41] focuses on the negative effects that screen-viewing is having on today's kids. In addition to increased tics as a potential reaction to screen use, she notes a higher incidence of ADHD, reported sleep problems, behavioral difficulties, and high levels of stress in today's kids.

Dunckley's solution? She advocates a strict four-week "fast" from screen use to see how these issues, including tics and academic performance, may improve. She suggests that if you observe improvement on the fast, you can then decide on a plan to move forward, given that complete avoidance is difficult to achieve.

Her list of the many devices that can trigger problems reflects how inundated we are with these products: *iPads, iPods, iPod Touches, video games, tablets, e-readers, cell phones and smart phones (including older models), laptops, notebooks, desktop computers, television sets, and DVD players.* It also highlights what a challenge it can be to control children's access.

The negative effects, Dr. Dunckley says, are noted not only from the visual impact of screens, but from their electromagnetic radiation as well.

She recommends these devices be removed from a child's bedroom, from cars, and from video game consoles in the home, including Wii and educational electronic games.

Reset Your Child's Brain features the case of Evan, a 10-year-old boy with tics. Evan was bright, yet socially awkward, and he experienced some attention difficulties. His parents allowed him to play video games and surf the internet for long hours at a time. They noted, though, that his tics would "go crazy" at these times.

Dr. Dunckley recommended to Evan's parents that they remove his access to electronics. She was sure there would be a big improvement because he was spending so much time in those activities. However, after two months, the parents reported that there had not been much change in the tics. Surprised at the lack of change, Dr. Dunckley then encouraged them to see what screen sources they might be overlooking.

Soon it was discovered that the boy had two "hidden" exposures to screens: an old laptop under his bed, and access to video games when visiting at the home of a relative. Once those screen options were eliminated, the parents found that Evan was happier, more organized, and that he turned in more homework. Plus, his tics were negligible.

Screens are only one of many environmental influences that surround us every day. They are a special challenge for families to monitor and control due to their popularity and widespread use.

Notes

_____

_____

_____

_____

_____

_____

_____

_____

_____

_____

_____

_____

_____

_____

_____

_____

_____

The ethics of ignoring triggers for tics

The physician's Hippocratic Oath: "First, do no harm"

If we visit a doctor with ongoing complaints of, for example, foot or chest pain, recurring stomach aches, lightheadedness, or difficulty breathing, we can expect that an effort will be made to determine what is causing the problem.

But, if your complaint is tics? A short checklist is used to assign a label to the type of tics being experienced (see pages 8-9). While some conditions may be ruled out, the patient is usually sent home with no effort made to learn what is actually *causing* the abnormal movements or vocalizations.

Not only is this approach not helpful, but it can be harmful. Specifically, when triggers are involved, it means that exposures to the same allergic, dietary, and/or toxic influences that played a role in bringing a person to the doctor in the first place are likely to continue.

Imagine you start sneezing 100 times a day. Red flags go up and a medical inquiry starts with the goal of finding out what could possibly be triggering the unusual sneezing. Yet, a person can holler uncontrollably 100 times a day, or jerk his or her neck 100 times a day, and that individual is often advised:

- "Sorry, but this is a genetic problem. There is nothing you can do about it."

- "Don't worry, your child will probably outgrow it."
- "Well, you can expect that the tics will wax and wane, come and go—we don't really know why."
- "If your tics continue for a year it might be Tourette syndrome."
- "Try to reduce stress. If the tics do not go away, let's talk about medications."

Not only is the cause not explored, but drugs with the potential for serious side effects are introduced.

This approach has been the status quo for so long that it is not questioned by mainstream medicine. Yet, surely physicians wish they had better options to offer their patients–effective and safer ways to improve symptoms.

Given that the treatment for tics is widely recognized as being unsatisfactory, it is unconscionable to ignore the possible role of tic triggers. Understanding how they can impact tics offers needed and realistic hope for symptom improvement. For one person, trigger knowledge may provide the key answers he or she needs. For another, it may prove to at least be part of the answer, allowing for less reliance on conventional therapies.

Not everyone will be interested in looking for triggers, and some who search may not find or be able to avoid them. But in any event, the concept is grounded in common sense. An effort to identify dietary, allergic, and environmental triggers is an accepted and important practice in many health conditions, and it should be considered for tic disorders as well.

Here is a snapshot of conventional tic treatment

Haloperidol (Haldol), pimozide (Orap), and aripiprazole (Abilify) are presently FDA approved medications to treat tics. Each of these is an antipsychotic and has the potential for significant, dangerous side-effects.

- Antipsychotic drugs are sometimes prescribed to children as young as three years of age. These medications are notorious for their serious potential side effects, some of which can be permanent. Along with other possible negative effects, these include dystonia (a term for continuous spasms and muscle contractions); muscle rigidity; tremors; severe anxiety; suicidal ideation; and even death.

- A range of other types of medications include, in part, central adrenergic inhibitors, antidepressants, and anti-seizure drugs. Generally, these also have the potential for unwanted side effects, although they are considered safer (while often less effective) than antipsychotics.

- Deep-brain stimulation via electrodes implanted in the brain may be offered to adults and teens with severe tics that do not respond to medications. Potential side-effects of deep-brain stimulation include seizure, infection, serious behavioral changes, confusion, stroke, and complications with the hardware used.

According to a 2017 report in *Parkinson's News Today*, surgical costs for deep-brain stimulation can run as high as $65,000 per patient, with battery replacements adding $10,000 - $20,000 to the cost over the first three years.

A *sad fact*: Keep in mind that the option of deep-brain stimulation is considered after trials of medications have failed. These medications would no doubt include at least one of the FDA approved antipsychotics. As noted above, these powerful drugs *can create* disabling and permanent spasms, tremors and muscle rigidity—a situation which may then lead to the invasive surgical option of deep-brain stimulation.

Comprehensive behavioral intervention for tics is promoted as an approach to avoid drug therapy. (See page 12). This intervention can be beneficial for some people and does not have detrimental physical side-effects. Yet why should someone go through the training and ongoing process of changing their habits without being aware that diet, allergy, or toxic exposures might be involved in their symptoms? Avoidance of these types of triggers could potentially eliminate the need for training and daily practice, or serve to complement the effort.

Do you remember reading about these cases?

- A young boy's tics were so bad that he had to walk on all fours. (Page 65-66)

- While growing up, a man's Tourette's was so severe that he was socially isolated. Medications were not helpful, and it made his father cry. (Page 50-53)

- A girl could not read because her neck kept jerking back, and her hands ripped pages out of her book. (Pages 58-59)

- A man had tried 14 psychiatric drugs to control tics, some of which made symptoms worse. Tics were tormenting him when, as an adult, he found his trigger answers. (Pages 95-96)

- A child developed four or five types of tics at once. She cried because her shoulder hurt from the relentless arm jerking, and vocal tics included animal-like sounds. (Pages 63-64)

- A boy could not feed himself because he could not control his hands. At times he could not speak due to the tics, and the parents described it as gut-wrenching to watch. (Page 57-58)

In each of these cases, as well as in other reports in this book, symptoms were eliminated or improved by the identification and avoidance of triggers.

We must ask: How can it possibly be ethical to prescribe dangerous drugs or perform deep-brain neurosurgery to reduce tics, when potential triggers for symptoms have not even been discussed with a patient, much less professionally explored?

Leaders in the field need to be held accountable

Genetic research is valuable, and the development of safe and effective drugs for tics would be a welcomed milestone. Yet, at the patient level, positive impact from these efforts remains a future promise.

After being involved in this field for 25 years, I have accumulated proof of the role that medical politics has played in stifling awareness of the role of dietary, allergic, and environmental tic triggers.

It is a very basic concept: If you want to solve a mystery, you have to examine all the clues. Yet, when physicians, patients, and family members have shared reports of tic triggers with the powerful medical board of the Tourette Association of America (Tourette Syndrome Association) there has not been responsible follow-up. This organization is singled out because it is the most influential voice in the field, and it is also the most heavily funded, with an annual budget of several million dollars. I also know for a fact that they are well aware of the efforts of ACN (*Latitudes.org*).

Busy clinicians cannot be expected to keep up with the thousands of new studies and journal reports published each year. It is the "opinion leaders" who filter information to doctors and help develop best practices for prevention, diagnosis, and treatment. These leaders should be held accountable for failing to share vital information with practitioners, and for failing to promote research focused on environmental, allergic, and dietary influences in tic disorders.

The public deserves answers to these questions:

- Published studies support a link between allergy and tics. When will the public and medical community learn of this connection so they can explore a possible link for themselves? When will additional research in this area be encouraged?

- When will protocols for the prevention and treatment of tics include the fact that synthetic additives in the diet can potentially trigger tics, just as they have been proven to trigger symptoms for some other conditions, including ADHD?

- When will people be warned that exposures to common environmental chemicals like gas fumes, exhaust, pesticides, perfumes/fragrances, air fresheners, VOCs, herbicides, formaldehyde, and chlorine can potentially exacerbate tics?

- When will it be common knowledge that food intolerance and food allergy can play a role in some people's tics, just as diet impacts many other medical conditions?

What lies behind the narrow-minded approach to tics?

Renowned nutritional expert, Dr. Abram Hoffer (1917–2009), told me during an interview: "In general, it takes two generations for new ideas to be accepted, perhaps even 50 years in medicine because of the huge monolithic medical establishment that has one mission: to preserve its own territory."

Is this what has been preventing progress? Does this explain why those in the field of neurology, psychology, and psychiatry seem reluctant to collaborate with specialists in other disciplines that appear to hold some of the answers to tic disorders? These disciplines include, in part, allergy and immunology, gastroenterology, endocrinology, toxicology, environmental medicine, and nutritional medicine.

One of our members suggested another motive, quoting the author Upton Sinclair: "It is difficult to get a man to understand something when his salary depends upon his not understanding it."

Some have further pointed to the pervasive and insidious influence of the food and drug industry.

I leave it to others to sort out the motivations that have resulted in patients and families being left in the dark about potential triggers for tics.

Whatever excuses may be offered, they are indefensible. The number of children, teens, and adults suffering from Tourette syndrome and related tic conditions keeps increasing, while leaders wait . . . for what?

The suppression of information on tic triggers—as has occurred in this field—is not only unethical. It is harmful and cruel.

Section Four

Tricky triggers

After identifying triggers

10

Tricky triggers

Sometimes you get lucky in your search. You might, just as an example, reduce sugars and remove synthetic additives from the diet and find that tics improve dramatically. Or, you might connect the dots and realize that tics started up when allergy season began, or after starting kitchen renovations that released formaldehyde or other toxins into the air. However, it typically takes some trial and error to come up with the answers you need.

For getting started quickly with foods, allergist Dr. Doris Rapp suggests you list the top five favorite foods and two favorite beverages. Then, stop consuming everything containing ingredients in these foods for a week or more to see if symptoms improve. If so, then add them back, one at a time over a number of days, to see whether that helps pinpoint specific causes of food-related symptoms.

Influences from different types of trigger sources may occur at the same time. In these situations, logging your observations can be essential. Keep in mind that foods are rarely eaten in isolation. We often consume a few or more items at the same meal, with several ingredients within a given dish or product. Let us say you notice that tics increased after breakfast. Well, what specifically was bothersome? If it is not clear to you, it is best to document each item, including the ingredients, so you can cross-reference later when you have time to compare foods and symptom changes. (Consider noting whether the item was or was not organic.) Also, write down any special events or environmental exposures that occurred. See Chapter 12 for information about accessing useful logs on our *Latitudes.org/trigger-resources* webpages.

Similarly, if there is an increase in tic symptoms after eating pizza, you should examine: Was it the wheat and/or something in the crust, like yeast or dough conditioner? Was it tomato or something else in the sauce? Was it a seasoning? Cheese? Added toppings? The answer is not always easy to tease out, but it can be done, and having a good log will help.

Keep an open mind during this process. And, do not assume that because others report that something affected their case that these same items will apply to you.

Some people initially zero in on items that are often reported as triggers, not just for tics, but for other conditions such as ADHD and autism. Casein (in milk) and gluten are frequently targeted. The fact is, for some people, avoidance of foods containing gluten and/or casein is an important key to their success in reducing tic symptoms. Yet for others, these dietary restrictions are not required. Just as one youngster can eat peanut butter every day, while a minuscule amount of the same food will have tragic consequences for a small percentage of others, we are all biologically different.

When triggers get complicated: PANDAS, PANS, and more

Some situations can confound trigger hunts. When a person is exceptionally fatigued, anxious, or has an illness, a potential trigger will typically be more bothersome than when the same exposure occurs while rested, healthy, and calm. Similarly, circumstances like being in the middle of an allergy season, or being overloaded with other troublesome exposures, can make some people more reactive at one time than another.

The difference in response levels during a variety of scenarios can often be confusing, possibly causing you to question if an item really is a trigger, even when it is—and vice versa. The answer for this possibility is to watch for a pattern over time.

Infections can affect gut health and, in turn, make someone more prone to food and immune reactions. Also, a viral, parasitic, or bacterial infection has the potential to create brain inflammation, with tics as one of the consequences. As an example, Lyme disease, caused by a bacterium transmitted from ticks, can cause symptoms that are sometimes misdiagnosed as Tourette syndrome.

PANDAS is an acronym for a childhood condition known as pediatric autoimmune neuropsychiatric disorder associated with streptococcus. This condition is an autoimmune response to strep that causes inflammation in the brain. PANDAS was defined in 1998 by Dr. Susan Swedo and colleagues. The diagnostic criteria has evolved since then. In this condition, distressing changes come on suddenly and can include severe obsessions and compulsions or tics, along with a combination of fears, separation anxiety, sensory sensitivities, mood swings, immature behavior or talk, an eating disorder, hyperactivity, sudden bedwetting, and/or loss of academic skills. Symptoms can be so intense as to be debilitating.

With time it was learned that different types of infections could also trigger these symptoms. In other words, the immune response was not restricted to strep. At this point, PANS (pediatric acute-onset neuropsychiatric syndrome) was defined. PANDAS is a subset of PANS.

PANS is a complex medical condition that requires expert evaluation and intervention. A full discussion is beyond the scope of this book. Antibiotics, antivirals, or antifungals are the first line of defense, depending on the nature of the infectious trigger. In some cases, IVIG (intravenous immunoglobulin) treatment and/or plasmapheresis are used to address the abnormal and misdirected immune response. Early identification is important.

There is considerable controversy within the medical and scientific community related to best practices for the diagnosis and treatment of PANS. Some practitioners actually refuse to accept the concept of PANS, and beyond that, approaches can vary between doctors. To stay abreast of research, check the website *pandasnetwork.org*. Also, the PANDAS/PANS forum on *Latitudes.org* offers support and cutting-edge ideas for dealing with these conditions.

According to guidelines, a diagnosis of PANS should rule out classic OCD, anorexia, Tourette syndrome, Sydenham chorea, transient tic disorder, bipolar disorder, and autoimmune encephalitis, among other more rare conditions. A conclusion from a PANS Collaborative Consortium (2013) was that, while referral to a neurologist or rheumatologist can be helpful, these "subspecialists may not be experienced with the evaluation of psychiatric symptomatology." It was suggested that the responsibility of evaluating PANS should fall to primary care clinicians and child psychiatrists. The full report is available for free online. Search for "Recommendations from the 2013 PANS Consensus Conference" to learn more.[42] Search also for an update: "Revised Treatment Guidelines Released for Pediatric Acute Onset Neuropsychiatric Syndrome (PANS/PANDAS)" (July 2017).

Our organization's publication *Your Child Has Changed: Should You Consider PANDAS?* offers a primer for families on this disorder.

When dealing with PANS, Lyme, or other infections, we recommend that, while pursuing medical treatment, families should be vigilant for dietary, allergic, and environmental triggers and practice avoidance for any identified. It is not unusual to observe a heightened response to triggers during this time.

The challenge of dealing with "masking"

The phenomenon of masking can complicate finding triggers. Masking means that your body has done its best to adapt to a personally harmful item, whether a food, allergen, or toxin. Chronic symptoms such as, for example, fatigue, digestive complaints, tics, or headache may occur but the person does not associate the symptom(s) with a particular item because they are exposed to it on a regular basis.

If you drink diet soda often and wonder if it is aggravating your tics, simply drinking a larger amount of the soda one day would not be expected to reveal much. Instead, you should "unmask" yourself to it by avoiding the soda(s) for several days. Then, test by consuming the diet soda to see if it triggers symptoms and is a problem.

Dr. Claudia Miller explains on her website (*DrClaudiaMiller.com/about-tilt*) that dealing with masking is particularly difficult once a person has become sensitized to numerous triggers.

While masking can be a challenge, it is not an insurmountable obstacle. Many people have found their tic triggers by being aware of this principle, and it is the concept behind elimination diets. When needed, consult an environmental physician or allergist for help with the process.

Cast a wide net when troubleshooting

When you start to brainstorm what might be contributing to tics, look at all the circumstances that could be playing a role. Avoid the temptation to focus only on food, for example. And, when thinking of toxins or allergens, look beyond your own familiar home setting. Explore what other locations might be involved.

One approach you can take is to print a copy of the lists of possible triggers in Chapter 7. Then, cross out all the ones you clearly know are not an issue. As an example, a child does not drink alcohol, so you would cross off that potential trigger. See what you are left with. Then, narrow the list to the ones that you think are most likely to be possibilities in your case and circle those.

It is sometimes useful to talk things through with someone else as you pinpoint areas on which to focus. Follow this up with use of the logs (see Chapter 12). While the process does require being a detective, few things are more rewarding than finding answers.

Level the playing field before you begin

There is no proven right or wrong approach to finding tic triggers. But, it can be helpful to put some basic conditions in place before you begin your search. Outlined here, these steps are relatively easy to accomplish and can be a practical starting point.

Of course, you may have a family history that sends you in a certain direction for your search, or your observations may have already provided clues that encourage you to use a particular approach. This is fine. Further, some people decide to "jump in with both feet" and initially explore every possibility they can think of that might be involved with symptoms. This all-at-once approach is often used by people dealing with serious tics who are anxious to find relief as soon as possible; they know that later they can always try to determine which specific factors are the most relevant.

The following preliminary steps are recommended as a starting point because it is possible that one or more of these issues may be having a major impact on tics. If you do not address these in advance, you could end up trying a number of different time-consuming efforts, when these adjustments themselves might have helped.

In addition, if any of these are significant triggers in your case and exposures to them continue, it will be more difficult for you to tease out other potentially important influences.

Preliminary steps:

- Eliminate foods with caffeine, artificial flavors, colors, and preservatives. Read labels and try to be strict and consistent.

- Make a note now of any foods that, based on previous observations, you suspect might be aggravating tics. Plan to avoid them.

- Cut way back on sugary foods and do not use artificial sweeteners like Nutrasweet/Equal.

- Replace chemically-scented products in the home with natural, unscented products.

- Create an allergy-free bedroom.

- Reduce/limit television viewing, video games, and screen time throughout the day.

- Eat organic when you can, and drink purified water.

After a couple of weeks with these efforts, make a note if you see tics reduce in frequency or severity. Once your hunt for triggers is underway, continue with the above suggestions.

Working with logs

First, give yourself a pat on the back if you are willing to keep a log for diet, exposures, symptoms, and any special occurrences that might affect tics, like a stressful situation, illness, or spending time in a new location.

We have developed several different types of logs, specific to tics, to help you. They are highlighted in Chapter 12 along with recommendations for use. You can download these free printable charts from our resources webpages at: *Latitudes.org/trigger-resources.*

You can also explore using different types of logs or apps offered by other companies and organizations, such as those for tracking weight-loss or migraine, and adapt them for your use. The key is to regularly document what is happening, even when you do not think something may be important at the time.

After identifying triggers

Once triggers for tics are determined, the next step is to decide what you are going to do about them. For example:

- A man may find that his companion's cologne or perfume bothers him, but he doesn't want to admit to having chemical sensitivities.

- Spouses or family members may have different levels of conviction about the need to make changes around the home to address toxins or allergens. One could be eager to begin modifications while the other is not motivated to pursue adjustments or does not believe they will make a difference.

- Parents may notice that certain favorite foods affect their child's symptoms. But, they do not want to upset the youngster by withholding these items, especially when the child already has to deal with having tics.

Be prepared that these are all classic types of issues you may find you need to work through.

When it comes to kids and diet, it is natural to want to make a child happy. But caregivers need to understand that a child with a tic disorder has a nervous system that is out of balance. For a number of possible reasons, he or she is hypersensitive or hyperexcitable. The goal needs to be to make the nervous system healthier and less reactive. If select foods are upsetting the balance, then diet issues need to be addressed. Naturally you want to avoid upsetting a child and you do not want to create undue stress. But do your best to set a goal and stick with it, with the long-term interests of the child at heart. Aim to find safe substitute items and have them available whenever you can. The rewards can outweigh the needed effort.

Some people may be able to deal with an occasional dietary lapse without a significant reaction; it all depends on the circumstances. But for others, there might be a severe response to a small exposure. In this case, continued exposure will be harmful. If indeed something that can be controlled is making symptoms worse, then it is important that it be avoided when feasible.

Clearly, we all make health-related decisions for ourselves every day related to diet, exercise, and lifestyle in general. In the same way that some adults may decide that they would rather deal with certain tics than experience the side effects of tic medications, they may also decide to continue indulging in a particular habit that they know aggravates their tics. That is their call. A child, however, should ideally be provided with the most wholesome environment feasible, and this responsibility falls to the caregiver(s). This includes diet, as well as avoiding toxins and allergens, trying to ensure adequate sleep, and providing emotional support.

Finding your balance point

A fellow recently approached me at a conference. He explained that he had experienced tics for many years, but during a trip to Europe he observed a significant reduction in symptoms. He realized the food he ate while there was much less processed than his typical diet in the U.S.A. Processed food products often have added chemicals and/or hydrogenated, cheap fats, with less nutrition than unadulterated foods. His tics were so improved that it inspired him to focus on unprocessed foods once back home. He also eliminated dairy and grains. The diet change made a dramatic difference in reducing his tics.

I spoke with this man by phone the following month and asked how he was doing. He said that while he knows the diet helps him, he really (really!) loves food. He decided on a "happy medium" approach, for which he avoids most of his trigger foods but still enjoys some off-diet items at times, resulting in mild tics that he feels he can live with.

Keep in mind that it tends to be easier for people to stick with a diet, or deal with environmental adjustments such as using unscented personal products, when others in the family are following the same plan.

As we know, parents do not have full control over what children eat or do throughout the day. As kids get older, they will want to make more of their own decisions on how they approach triggers. Of course, when they eventually leave home for college or to live on their own, all bets are off. It is normal for them to assert their independence. If triggers have been identified, they will balance the social ramifications of having tics with the adjustments they are willing to make. Motivations will vary based on the severity of tics, the effort needed to implement change, the benefits they have (or have not) experienced with tic trigger avoidance, peer issues, and changing personal circumstances. Try to remain supportive and accepting during this time.

Keep an eye out for the unexpected

It would be misleading to suggest that all tic symptoms for all people can be controlled simply by changing the diet or the immediate environment. In some cases, a significant health or emotional issue can override typical adjustments you may try to make. This does not mean that avoiding triggers is not important; strive to do so whenever practical while also addressing other needs.

For the chemically sensitive, ongoing awareness is needed outside the home to avoid pollution, pesticides, and allergic influences. A golf course or athletic field may look green and fresh, but it could be loaded with newly applied herbicides and pesticides. A remodeled work space at the office might be long overdue, but be aware that new carpeting, paint, and furniture might outgas (release) toxins.

A daycare room may look sparkling clean, yet might have been cleaned with harsh chemicals, and/or may have pest control products applied in walls, cracks, and crevices. Heading to the grandparents' home can be a good getaway, but if Grandma wears perfume, Grandpa smokes, or the home is moldy with sugary, processed snacks in the cupboard, the visit might spell trouble.

As an example of how insidious toxic exposures can be, in the book *Child Health and the Environment*,[43] a chapter on pesticides includes information on automatic insecticide dispensers registered by the EPA for use in restaurants, schools, supermarkets, daycare centers, and other facilities to control indoor flying insects.

These can be set to dispense a fine mist as often as every 15 minutes, or as programmed. Although recommendations are made for off-hour use, and safety precautions are provided with the device, there is little oversight of their actual use. And, chances are you will not even know they are there. Similarly, auto-mist devices are used in public places to spray air fresheners that often contain toxins.

Learn what the environmental policies are for your places of work, in your community, and in schools. Get involved when needed. Your questions and discussions will help educate others. A number of online resources give pointers for dealing with these issues. And remember, tics are not the only detrimental health consequence of toxic and allergic exposures.

Avoid what you can, and be proactive in your home setting—the one area you can best control.

Using incentive charts to encourage new habits

Regardless of age, diet change is not always easy and rarely popular. No one likes to have limits imposed when it comes to enjoying food. Adults are usually mature enough to weigh the pros and cons of making adjustments to their eating habits. Gaining compliance from children, however, is a goal and not a given.

To help in this effort with kids, ACN (*Latitudes.org*) has colorful, free printable sticker and reward charts in PDF format, many of which can be used to encourage compliance and sustain enthusiasm. These can be easily downloaded and printed for use. Premium subscription members of ACN have the option to fill in text fields for charts online before printing, to avoid the necessity of writing by hand.

See Chapter 12 for information on charts we have developed specifically for trigger searches, including tools for adolescents and adults.

Be sure to provide verbal support to those who are adapting to change, whether for dietary issues or other factors. Acknowledge how difficult, but worthwhile, it can be to make whatever adjustments are on your agenda. Limiting activities where there is exposure to toxins, such as a swimming pool or an herbicide-treated playing field, takes special consideration when dealing with a chemically sensitive child.

Communicate with teachers, friends, and family so you can win support and hopefully achieve consistency in your plans. Specialty or restricted diets are much more common these days than in the past, and that is a plus.

Getting to the root cause of sensitivities

I often encourage anyone dealing with tics to think of twitches, jerks, and vocalizations as symptoms of an underlying illness or physical imbalance. It is not unusual for patients with a tic disorder to also experience one or more health complaints such as aches and pains, cramps, "feeling sick," and/or sensitivity to heat, touch, or light. Digestive issues, migraine and headaches, night terrors, problems falling asleep and waking, bed-wetting, talking during sleep, visual defects, and vomiting are also common issues among those with a diagnosis of Tourette syndrome.

While avoiding triggers whenever you can, it is good to think holistically. Encourage your physician to fully explore *all* the symptoms that are being experienced, not just the tics. Request a referral to a specialist to address these issues, when needed. Do not overlook the possibility of an unidentified, underlying infection.

In addition to exploring allergic status and diet, consider looking into possible biochemical imbalances, toxic overloads requiring a detoxification approach, a candida overload in the digestive tract, physical asymmetry that may be exerting abnormal pressure on nerves, and a need for nutrient supplementation. In *Natural Treatments for Tic and Tourette's: A Patient and Family Guide*, medical specialists give recommendations on strategies to address health problems that can accompany or result in tics.

It is often possible to strengthen the immune system and improve resilience, with the result that some previous triggers are no longer as troublesome as they initially were. Efforts to strengthen the immune system, or reduce the level of stress response in your body, can require professional assistance. I encourage you to seek the help you need.

Tools in the next chapter are designed to support your efforts in identifying and dealing with tic triggers.

Section Five

Get help: Trigger Resources webpages

How you can help ACN's effort

Get help: Trigger-Resources webpages

Whether this is your first experience looking for triggers, or you are hoping to fine-tune approaches you have already made, you can find helpful tools on our special Trigger-Resources webpages. This free online feature has been developed for you as a supplement to this book.

www.Latitudes.org/trigger-resources

- The charts and logs described on upcoming pages can be downloaded from this resource.

- Links are given for additional information and to assist you in finding professional help

I hope some of these tools will benefit you during your journey as you seek to identify and avoid tic triggers.

After many years of providing material for members of ACN: *Latitudes.org,* we know that people often take advantage of charts and logs like those in this chapter to help them begin a dialogue with loved ones, keep their efforts fresh, and document new plans and ideas.

Completed forms provide a rich source of information that can be used to analyze or jump-start your endeavors whenever you wish. While some readers will find they do not need the support of logs and charts, others may even build on the ideas in this chapter and develop their own methods. I wish everyone the very best in finding what fits their unique situation.

Daily Log for Tic Triggers

Daily Log for Tic Triggers

Name_____   Date_____

Symptoms on waking _____

_____

_____

_____

_____

Breakfast _____

_____

_____

_____

_____

Symptoms after breakfast _____

_____

_____

_____

_____

Morning snack _____

_____

_____

_____

Lunch_____

_____

_____

_____

_____

Afternoon symptoms_____

_____

_____

_____

_____

Afternoon snack_____

_____

_____

_____

Dinner/Late snack _____

_____

_____

_____

_____

Symptoms before bed_____

_____

_____

_____

*Toxic or allergic exposures, medications, amount
of screen time, activities, illness, special circumstances*

_____

_____

_____

_____

_____

_____

_____

_____

*Comments*_____

_____

_____

_____

_____

Overall tic level   1   2   3   4   Overall behavior   1   2   3   4

A supplement to *Tourette Syndrome: Stop Your Tics by Learning What Triggers Them* (c) ACN Latitudes.org

Download in full-size from www.Latitudes.org/trigger-resources

DAILY LOG FOR TIC TRIGGERS

The "Daily Log for Tic Triggers" is designed for you to record dietary, environmental and other influences, along with tic symptoms. When kept carefully for the purposes of a trigger search, it can yield valuable information. It is a good idea to print several sheets at a time so you have them readily on hand.

Keep completed pages in a folder for comparison and future reference. A pattern connecting tics to items in the log might be revealed after a short amount of time, or you may need considerable patience before being able to identify anything that is associated with an increase in tic symptoms.

Short codes Plan to develop your own short codes for recording. For example, rather than writing out "vocal tics" you could just use V. And, if you repeat a certain food item or activity often, decide on an abbreviation to easily represent this. Remember though, that individual ingredients make a difference. So, if you routinely have toast at breakfast, unless you use the same bread and spread every day, simply putting "toast" will be incomplete. You need to specify the exact bread and spread used, or you could end up overlooking certain ingredients that have been playing a role in the tics. Please see the "Ingredients Reference" chart (page 136) if you want to document a given product just once to avoid having to record ingredients repeatedly.

Amounts Naturally, the *amount* of food and drink consumed makes a difference. Find a way to indicate if you had significantly more or less than the amount you would usually have. Remember, though, that the focus is not on calories—the goal is not weight loss or gain. Rather, you are focusing on whether an item is having an effect on the nervous system. If a serving of a particular juice is typically 8-ounces for you, then you could just record the specific type of juice without bothering to indicate the amount each time. But, let us say you have 3 glassfuls—or in contrast, just half a glass—consider adding 3x or 1/2, showing it was more or less than normal. In addition to this notation, you will have recorded what was contained in the juice.

Organic foods Avoiding pesticides is preferable for everyone's health. However, for someone with significant chemical sensitivities, non-organic food can directly exacerbate tics. Use a simple symbol to indicate the foods that were, or were not, organic.

Cumulative reactions Sometimes food sensitivities are cumulative. If you have a sensitivity (in contrast to an allergy) to dairy, for example, you might be able to get away with consuming some items with dairy for a couple of days, but then on a third day of having dairy you find tics are affected. Watch for this type of pattern when you review your logs.

Go beyond diet While food and drink are the most common types of triggers people focus on, be sure to expand your efforts and record other influences mentioned on this log. Changes in stress levels, emotional issues, medications, anxiety, chemical exposures, allergens, and other environmental factors, as well as types of activities, can all play a role. Take a few minutes each day to review these. *Note:* Screen time should be documented if this could be a factor in your situation.

Need more specifics? Depending on the complexity of your case, you may find you need to record additional details by jotting notes on the back of the log or attaching a separate sheet.

Over time, the recording will become easier and you will develop a greater ability to assess potential triggers, almost as second nature.

To fill the form online: If you wish, you can use Adobe Acrobat to open the PDF log file that you download from our Trigger-Resources page and complete it online each day. When finished, print it right away for your records, or, save it in an online folder. (Just be sure to "save" the document under a different file name each day, or you will record over your previous one.) As with the printed and handwritten version, keep the forms organized for future reference.

Checklist for Observing and Brainstorming Tic Triggers

Checklist for Observing and Brainstorming Tic Triggers

Keep this sheet handy so you can update it as you become aware of influences that may be affecting tics. Using a daily log as a companion effort can be very useful.

Location
___Generally worse indoors
___Generally worse outdoors
___Better at beach
___Better in countryside
___Worse in air conditioning
___Worse in a particular room of home
___Worse when in bed or on awakening
___Worse when heat turned on
___Worse in damp places or basements
___Worse in specific locations
___Worse in car (new ___ old ___)
___Worse after school bus ride
___Worse at gas station
___Worse on sports fields or golf courses
___Worse in stores with perfumes/candles
___Worse in certain types of lighting
___Worse in aisles with pest/lawn/laundry products
___Worse with home-remodeling, fresh paint
___Worse with plug-ins/air fresheners
___Worse with indoor fresh holiday trees
Other_____

Time/season/weather
___Worse in cold or ___heat
___Worse in fall season
___Worse in spring
___Worse in evening or ___morning
___Worse during or after rain
___Worse in bright sunlight
Other_____

Activities
___Worse when dusting or vacuuming
___Worse when using cleansers
___Worse when raking leaves or cutting grass
___Worse around dogs, cats, other animals
___Worse around smoke/smog/air pollution
___Worse after certain meals or foods
___Worse with certain clothing
___Worse with loud noises
___Worse when stressed, anxious, or excited
___Worse when tired or after exertion
___Worse with video gaming/television viewing
___Worse with computer/tablet use
___Worse when using hair products/scented soaps
___Worse with bug repellent
___Worse around odors
___Worse when using crafts, markers, paints
Other_____

Miscellaneous
___Worse or ___better after dental procedures
___Worse or ___better premenstrually
___Worse or ___better with allergy medication
___Worse or ___better with antibiotics
___Worse or ___better with steroids
___Worse or ___ better with viral/bacterial infection

Notes:
_____
_____
_____

Download in full-size from www.Latitudes.org/trigger-resources

CHECKLIST FOR OBSERVING AND BRAINSTORMING TIC TRIGGERS

Jog your memory and open your mind to possible triggers with this convenient checklist. As you read it through, chances are you will come across some situations or factors that you have not previously considered as possibly playing a role in your tic disorder. "Possibly" is the key term here. It would be expected that many of these items will not apply to your situation at all. Check-mark the ones you think could be the most relevant. Consider noting those you want to focus on in the coming days. Then, start to watch for cause-and-effect situations as you zero in on issues.

Consider clues Some of these items can help define a key problem. For example, if tics are worse when raking leaves, this could be indicative of a mold sensitivity, not simply a reaction to a particular type of tree(s) or grasses. Other red flags or clues for mold sensitivity would be if you checked the form for noticing a reaction to damp places or basements, and/or if you have noticed symptom increases after a rain. Give some thought to implications that might be associated with each item you check off.

Within your home If tics are worse in a certain room, focus on what sets that area apart from the others. The culprit might be linked to one or more issues such as, for example, a musty carpet or new laminate flooring, recent refurbishing, type of lighting, pet dander, scented deodorizers, electromagnetic radiation, air filters that need cleaning, heating or cooling issues, mold, dust, or other allergens. While the list may seem endless, it is not! Simply take your time to think through what makes that room "special."

It is advisable to revisit this "Checklist for Observing and Brainstorming Tic Triggers" form from time to time to see if your observations change.

Ingredient Reference

Once you have recorded ingredients for specific items consumed, save the form for easy reference in the future.

ITEM:

ITEM:

ITEM:

ITEM:

ITEM:

ITEM:

Download in color and full-size from www.Latitudes.org/trigger-resources

INGREDIENT REFERENCE

If nothing else convinces you to simplify your diet, this useful exercise may. As discussed previously, it is important to breakdown the ingredients in items you eat and drink so you can narrow down what might be aggravating tics. Just knowing the type of food is not sufficient. (Such as "salad").

Once you have recorded the ingredients for a specific item, then in the future you will be able to just refer to the sheet to know what was in it. Often, though not always, the longer the list, the greater the chance that it contains synthetic additives that are best avoided.

If you are not familiar with reading labels, you will soon be aware of the difference between a simple product, such as organic sea salt potato chips that contain only three ingredients (i.e., organic potatoes, organic safflower oil, and sea salt), and typical sour cream and onion "flavored" chips that might have more than 15 ingredients, some of them hard to even pronounce.

You might prefer printing the ingredients from the "nutrition" section of the manufacturer's website.

Remember, once you have completed information on a product, it is easy to refer back without additional effort required.

My Focus for Today

my focus for today

DATE

TO-DO

PRIORITIES

FOODS TO AVOID

SHOPPING LIST

MEALS

B

L

S

D

NOTES

Download in color and full-size from www.Latitudes.org/trigger-resources

MY FOCUS FOR TODAY

Making a fresh start each day can help keep your efforts to reduce tics on track. Whether you are just beginning your trigger search, or things are well underway and you no longer need to use more detailed logs, this optional form can encourage you to keep things moving in a positive direction.

Highlight key targets that you want to focus on. This can include efforts to deal with allergies and avoidance of toxins, not only foods.

Make brief notes of any special items consumed for meals in the Breakfast, Lunch, Snack, and Dinner (B,L,S,D) shaded bars.

Trigger Food Plan

TRIGGER FOOD PLAN

Monitor throughout the week and start a fresh log every several days.

AVOID THIS WEEK

_____
_____
_____
_____
_____
_____
_____
_____

ON THE OKAY LIST!

_____
_____
_____
_____
_____
_____
_____
_____

NOT SURE YET

_____
_____
_____
_____
_____
_____
_____

FAVORITES ALLOWED

_____
_____
_____
_____
_____
_____
_____

"I hate when I think I'm buying organic vegetables and when I get home I find they're just regular donuts."

Source unknown

(c) www.Latitudes.org

Download in color and full-size from www.Latitudes.org/trigger-resources

TRIGGER FOOD PLAN

A key to success when pursuing tic triggers is to write your plans down rather than keep them swirling around in your head (or scribbled on numerous post-it notes). This document will assist you in keeping your thoughts and plans organized.

Each of the four categories is self-explanatory. You do not have to tackle everything at once, so use this form to specify what you want to focus on in the coming week. Those goals will probably change with time, based not only on your trigger observations, but also on what the circumstances are for the coming days. For example, if you are traveling, your expectations would probably change. If home life is more hectic than usual or someone is sick, you may find yourself making adjustments.

Once the page is completed it should assist you in decision-making through-out the week. Be prepared to customize plans for future efforts as you gain new insights throughout the process.

Weekly Food Log

Weekly Food Log

Week_____

	Breakfast	Lunch	Dinner	Snacks/drinks
Sunday				
Monday				
Tuesday				
Wednesday				
Thursday				
Friday				
Saturday				

(c) Latitudes.org

Download in color and full-size from www.Latitudes.org/trigger-resources

WEEKLY FOOD LOG

Depending on your situation and the stage of your trigger search, you may find that a chart like this meets your needs by giving a quick weekly overview.

Ways to use the log This versatile log can be helpful in a number of ways.

1. You can summarize what you consume during each day, or;

2. Make a note of what you intend to put on your menu for the coming week, or;

3. Highlight only what you ate/drank that you think might have been troublesome.

Document if you notice a worsening or improvement in symptoms on a particular day or time of day. You can indicate symptom change on the chart itself with a 1 - 5 scale, for example, or maintain a record of this separately.

Remember to save completed logs.

Here's What I Think
Makes My Tics Worse

Here's what I think makes my tics worse

- ☐ Feeling too hot or too cold
- ☐ Watching TV
- ☐ Riding in a car or bus
- ☐ Being hungry
- ☐ Playing sports
- ☐ Being nervous
- ☐ Feeling tired
- ☐ Working on the computer
- ☐ When I'm worried
- ☐ When I'm angry
- ☐ Being excited
- ☐ Smelling things like perfume
- ☐ Smelling bug spray

- ☐ When my allergies are bad
- ☐ When I have a cold
- ☐ When I feel sick to my stomach
- ☐ When I have pizza
- ☐ Swimming in a pool
- ☐ Playing with a pet
- ☐ Playing video games
- ☐ When I drink _____
- ☐ Being at school
- ☐ Being in _____'s house.
- ☐ When I eat sweet things
- ☐ Using a tablet or iPad
- ☐ When I eat out

Other things that bother me:

_____

_____

_____

_____

Name_____ Date_____

(c) Latitudes.org

Download in color and full-size from www.Latitudes.org/trigger-resources

HERE'S WHAT I THINK MAKES MY TICS WORSE

Designed for use with older children and teens, this custom ACN: *Latitudes. org* form serves vital purposes. It can increase a person's personal awareness of tic triggers while strengthening a child's sense of self-empowerment. It is also a convenient way to let parents know of influences that they may not have realized were affecting their son or daughter.

Expectations This is a voluntary form, and you should expect neither complete honesty nor full awareness on the part of the user. In fact, you cannot even insist that the log be carefully completed. It is very possible that the person filling the form has never given much thought to tic triggers, after being told by a doctor or support group advocate that nothing affects tics besides stress and fatigue. With this in mind, let the youngster complete it however he or she wishes, without pressure. Sometimes the approach taken will depend on how motivated one is to eliminate tics. That said, it can be a very useful exercise.

Honor the concept The concept of this chart is to have it function as a self-report, for which the person gives some thought to each item and tries to determine whether it has impacted tics. The main point is that rather than parents expressing what *they* think might be playing a role in the symptoms, responses come from the user.

The process of reviewing these factors can help youngsters develop the understanding that tic triggers exist for many other kids, and some of these issues might be playing a role in their case as well. If you need to talk it through and give a hint on occasion (or even read it aloud, when needed) that is okay. But encourage personal awareness.

Continued

Everyone is different Explain that each person's tic triggers can be different, and these are just possibilities. Also mention that some people might not find triggers, but it is worth thinking about them because when they are found and avoided, then tics can be reduced and will sometimes even disappear. And that is a good thing.

The benefit This exercise can be reassuring, letting someone know that he or she may have some control over the tics. That said, it is not unusual for the user to fail to check off items that are clearly affecting symptoms, in an effort to avoid having restrictions placed on them. This is human nature. Be understanding of this if you notice it happening, and discuss if needed.

Growing awareness After the form is completed, suggest that the youngster start to be more aware in the future of what might be making tics worse, and make it clear that you will do your best to help with any situation that is found to be troublesome. Also, mention that sometimes it is hard to be sure of what is affecting tics, and that it is good to keep an open mind. The form can be repeated at any time. Hopefully, through this exercise you will also learn more about how tics are viewed by your son or daughter.

Your own goals Meanwhile, you can proceed with your parental efforts related to triggers, such as changing dietary plans, adjusting the home environment, or reducing screen time, regardless of the responses to this form.

My Food Contract

MY FOOD CONTRACT

Start date: _____ End date: _____

I understand that I should not eat or drink:

_____

_____

_____

_____ .

When I follow this plan for _____ week(s) I will have this reward:

_____

_____

_____ .

If I do not follow this agreement then:

_____

_____

_____ .

Signed _____ _____

Date_____

(c) Latitudes.org; A supplement to Stop Your Tics by Learning What Triggers Them

Download in color and full-size from www.Latitudes.org/trigger-resources

FOOD AND OTHER FAMILY CONTRACTS

Parent-child contracts have the advantage of being straightforward and easy to execute. They are ideal for use when a child is able to demonstrate a significant degree of self-discipline without needing frequent reinforcement of the type provided with a daily sticker chart, for example.

Flexible uses Contracts are often used for homework agreements, completing chores around the house, or specific behaviors. *The contract on the previous page is dedicated to diet. You can also find a general contract on our Trigger-Resources pages that you can adapt as you wish.*

In the context of tic triggers, you might choose to focus on developing behaviors related to:

- Avoiding stressful situations known to aggravate tics
- Limiting screen time
- Consuming only foods/drinks that are not on an "avoid" list
- Engaging in positive behaviors you want to encourage

A clear agreement A successful contract needs to be clearly understood by both parties. In the beginning, a single issue should be focused on. If you want to work on reducing screen time—or getting to bed at a certain time—then specify exactly what the expectation is for that goal. For example, do not in the same contract add that you also want to see higher grades in math, or more help around the house without complaining. Keep one target in mind. (As time goes on, you may find you can add more than one goal.)

Once the contract is filled out and signed, review it orally to be sure that there are no misunderstandings. For the sake of clarity, it can be a good practice to have kids verbalize what they believe the contract details are.

Selecting a reward Rewards are only motivating when they are something a person wants. While this seems obvious, the importance of determining the right reward is often overlooked. It does not have to be monetary. Discuss the reward to be sure it is mutually agreed upon, with no ambiguity.

A negative consequence? Research shows that most kids respond best to positive rewards. But there may be times when a negative form of discipline is helpful. The contract allows for a negative consequence in the section that says, "If I do not follow this agreement then." But whether you need to use that part of the contract depends on your family dynamics and the situation at hand. Feel free to leave the section blank.

Time frame A single contract is often developed for a week or more at a time. Be sure the length of time is specified on the form and clearly understood. Generally, the main purpose of contracts such as this is to have a short-term intervention that results in a positive outcome. If you choose to repeat the exact same contract, you can simply adjust the time-frame dates at the top, and have the parent and child initial the form. But, if changes are being made to the contract agreement itself, plan on starting a fresh form.

Stick to the Right Foods Daily Chart

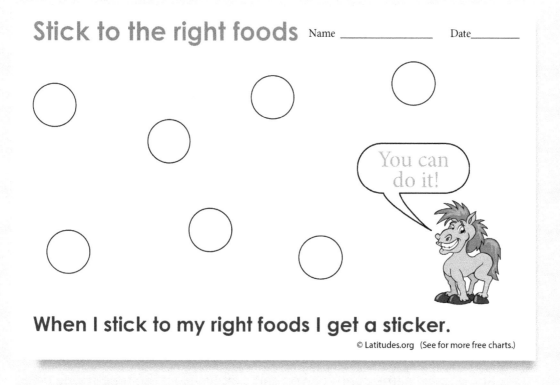

When I stick to my right foods I get a sticker.

© Latitudes.org   (See for more free charts.)

STICK TO THE RIGHT FOODS DAILY CHART

Sticker or incentive charts are a classic method of nudging behavior in a positive direction.

When trying to shape a young child's habits, frequent reinforcement is often needed, and this daily chart meets that need. Some kids do not require a chart like this. They readily comply with a parent's request and receive satisfaction in just knowing they did as requested: a smile, thank you, and words of support from Mom or Dad does the trick. Others, though, do better with a visual reminder and special recognition, and this can be accomplished through a sticker chart.

Rewarding with stickers When you print the "Stick to the Right Foods" PDF that you will download from *Latitudes.org/trigger-resources*, there will be two forms to a page. Typically you would use a half sheet each day, but some children may need a separate form for the morning and one for the afternoon because they require reinforcement often in order to keep them motivated and focused.

A variety of fun and colorful stickers for kids are readily available in school supply areas of stores, arts and crafts sections, scrapbooking stores, and even in the gift card section of many stores. If stickers are unavailable, you can always draw a smiley face.

As with any incentive chart, it is important to be clear on what is expected. Be sure to specify what you mean by "right foods." Review the plan with your child, writing down expectations on a separate sheet, or drawing examples, if needed.

In the context of tic triggers, you can reward with a sticker for eating or drinking an item (or consuming a full meal) that is on the dietary plan. But, you can also give a sticker for passing up something that is off limits: "You didn't eat the orange candy that Tonya offered you. Thank you. You just earned a sticker." Use of the sticker chart should be a positive experience for parent and child. Aim to completely fill the chart each day when a sincere effort is being made. The goal is to gain compliance.

Kids are different. Some will be proud to have the chart filled up, and no other reward is needed. Others may respond best if they earn a "ticket" or points for each completed sheet and when—just as an example—they have earned five tickets (or any number of points), they can stay up a little later, or pick the family TV movie to watch, have a friend over to play, take a trip to the library, etc. Agree on a simple reward for completing one or more charts.

Keep the chart focused When using this chart, stick to the issue of "right food." Whether or not children forget to feed the dog, beg for toys at the store, or squabble with a sibling, these types of behaviors do not factor into earning a sticker on this chart. Keep things focused on what the child actually ate and drank related to your diet plan.

Let us say you want to do a trial of no-dairy for two weeks. You might say something at breakfast like, "You had almond milk on your cereal and a pear instead of yogurt. Great. Pick two stickers and put them on the chart." Or at snack time: "Carrots with hummus instead of cheese—yes! Pick a sticker." If you have empty circles at the end of the day, make an effort to find excuses to fill the chart. "No glass of milk at dinner or at bedtime—two stickers." If dairy is consumed, either on purpose or by mistake, there is no punishment. As a general rule, do not remove stickers. But, if the child went off the diet plan intentionally, you can make sure the chart is not fully filled for that day, and talk about it. Emphasize any good effort that is being made as well.

Children's response to rewards So many factors play a role in approaching dietary change that flexibility is needed with incentive plans. As a matter of principle, parents may feel they do not want to have to "buy" compliance—yet on a daily basis, parenting is all about giving and withholding praise or other forms of reinforcement.

Children who need to face the challenge of going beyond the norm with their eating habits can thrive with a suitable, simple reward along with the extra attention that a chart naturally brings to the situation. Be prepared to switch to different designs to keep interest high. In most cases, incentive charts do not need to be used long-term.

For additional tips on successful uses of sticker charts and other incentive tools, and for ways to determine rewards that are inexpensive but actually work well, read *Behavior Charts to the Rescue!* which is available in the store on *Latitudes.org,* or on Amazon in Kindle format. It is loaded with helpful ideas and techniques.

Kids' Weekly Point or Sticker Charts

My food today
Week_____

	Breakfast	Lunch
SUNDAY		
MONDAY		
TUESDAY		
WEDNESDAY		
THURSDAY		
FRIDAY		
SATURDAY		

How I Did with Food Today
Week_____

	Breakfast	Lunch	Dinner	Snacks/drinks
Sunday				
Monday				
Tuesday				
Wednesday				
Thursday				
Friday				
Saturday				

(c) Latitudes.org

Download in color and full-size from www.Latitudes.org/trigger-resources

KIDS' WEEKLY POINT OR STICKER CHARTS

For these charts, you can award a single sticker for each cell when the child complies with the dietary expectations for that meal or snack. You can decide on a small reward for a total number of stickers in the week, or give daily incentives.

Do not expect perfection. A child should be able to obtain a reward without having a perfect sheet. Be flexible and do your best to make it a mutually enjoyable experience.

What Makes Me Tic?

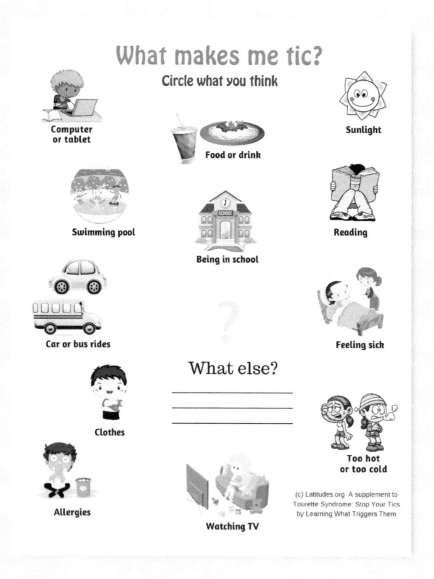

WHAT MAKES ME TIC?

This colorful chart for young children can best be used with someone who is already aware of his or her tics. When children are oblivious or completely unconcerned about their tics, it is usually best to ignore the topic and postpone introducing this chart until later. In this situation, there is no need to bring tics to the attention of the child.

Talk it through Once aware of ticcing, a youngster can benefit from this approach. It is designed to foster a better understanding of daily things that may be making tics worse. The chart can be used to start a discussion about how other families have found that one or more of the pictures on the paper have bothered other kids who have also tics. Explain that if something is making his or her tics worse, then, as a family, you will work together to help make things better.

Walk him or her through each picture and explain the image when needed. Talk about the "what else" section, and offer to fill it in for the child.

Moving ahead After your son or daughter has used the chart for the first time, encourage watching to see if anything new can be learned.

Plan to print a few copies to have on hand, and revisit the exercise from time to time. Some parents like to make special notes on the back of the sheet. Be sure to save completed forms in a safe place.

PANDAS/PANS Timeline

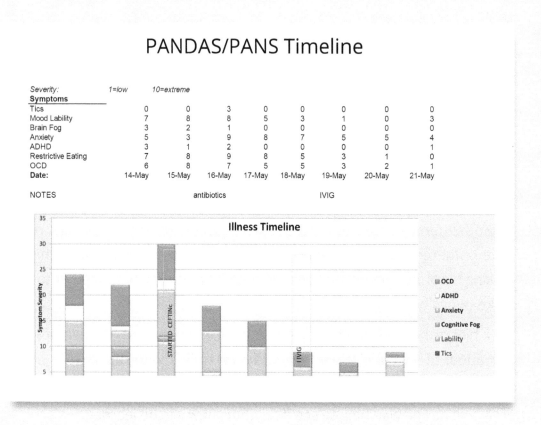

PANDAS/PANS Timeline

Severity:	1=low	10=extreme						
Symptoms								
Tics	0	0	3	0	0	0	0	0
Mood Lability	7	8	8	5	3	1	0	3
Brain Fog	3	2	1	0	0	0	0	0
Anxiety	5	3	9	8	7	5	5	4
ADHD	3	1	2	0	0	0	0	1
Restrictive Eating	7	8	9	8	5	3	1	0
OCD	6	8	7	5	5	3	2	1
Date:	14-May	15-May	16-May	17-May	18-May	19-May	20-May	21-May

NOTES   antibiotics   IVIG

Illness Timeline

Legend: OCD, ADHD, Anxiety, Cognitive Fog, Lability, Tics

Y-axis: Symptom Severity (5–35)

STARTED CEFTINC

IVIG

PANDAS/PANS TIMELINE CHART

The concept for this online chart was developed by a member of ACN: *Latitudes.org* who encountered major difficulties trying to track her child's variety of symptoms and numerous treatments/triggers related to PANDAS. (See about PANDAS/PANS on page 114-116.)

Using Microsoft Excel While other charts in this section can be printed as PDF documents, this chart requires a computer program such as Microsoft Excel. You will want to adapt the chart to meet your needs. One of the benefits of an Excel chart is that the details recorded can easily be converted to a graph, as shown. If you would like to track symptoms and treatments in this way but are not familiar with how to use a program like this, you can look for a tutorial on YouTube, or ask acquaintances to suggest someone who might volunteer to help you get started. (Of course, nowadays many kids know how to set something up like this as well.)

Microsoft Excel is a program that needs to be purchased. However, there are free similar programs available online, and an internet search will bring them up.

Instructions

1. List relevant symptoms in the far left column of your Excel chart. Insert or delete rows as needed

2. Insert dates; these can be daily or weekly

3. Rate each symptom at the end of each day and record it

4. Highlight the relevant dates you want to chart, and select the "chart tool" to create a stacked chart

5. You can insert text boxes onto the chart to note important events, medications, and treatments

6. Click on the chart to print only the chart and not the supporting data

Simplified chart option Instead of listing all symptoms, you can rate each day from 1 to 10 (ten being awful) as an overall score.

The creator of the chart added: "What I find helpful about using an Excel format is that it is really useful when you have multiple symptoms, not just tics. It lets you quantify good days and bad, and potentially see patterns more quickly—or see spikes every 7th day, for example. This is roughly how we realized that weekends were always better for our daughter; symptoms were reduced when she was home from school."

13

How you can help this effort

Spread the word on social media

The tic community needs your efforts to get the word out on tic triggers and other natural approaches to symptoms. *Please:*

- Like us on Facebook (fb.com/acnlatitudes | fb.com/stopticstoday)
- Follow us on Pinterest (pinterest.com/acnlatitudes)
- Share news of our book with your friends on social media
- Share our Tourette syndrome articles (from *Latitudes.org*) with your friends on social media

Be a member of ACN (*Latitudes.org*)

We offer free *Latitudes.org* memberships, and we also have an inexpensive paid premium membership. This membership gives benefits to you, while supporting the Association for Comprehensive NeuroTherapy (ACN). Please consider being a premium member.

Donate

We are very much in need of financial support for the efforts of ACN at *Latitudes.org* and for our fundraising website *StopTicsToday.org.* Can you help? Please see **www.Latitudes.org/donate** or **www.StopTicsToday.org/donate**

More on the next page

CHAPTER THIRTEEN

Connect with the news media

Triggers for tics is a newsworthy issue. Let Sheila Rogers DeMare know if you can network with radio, television, newspapers, or other news outlets. Please contact her through *www.Latitudes.org/contact*

Share with your doctor and support groups

You can make a difference by sharing news of this book with others, along with any of your own observations about identified triggers. Request your doctor to put a note in your medical file (or your child's) documenting any triggers you discover.

Help develop research grants

Please let us know if you have skills in grant writing and can volunteer to write proposals. Send a note to *www.Latitudes.org/contact*.

Sign up for the Amazon Smile Program

If you use Amazon for purchases, their Smile program will automatically send a small percentage of your purchase to a nonprofit of your choice. The Association for Comprehensive NeuroTherapy is an accepted charity for this purpose. Just look for the Smile program on the Amazon site and select us! Every little bit counts.

*Any and all efforts you can make to help us in this mission
are much needed and will be greatly appreciated.*

Section Six

Appendix A: Food additives

Appendix B: Salicylates and tyramine

Appendix C: Migraine and headache triggers

Bibliography

References and additional reading
On tics and Tourette syndrome
On environmental and allergic issues: non-specific
On triggers for medical conditions including ADHD

Also

Publications from the Association
for Comprehensive NeuroTherapy

Appendix A: Food additives

Artificial colors

Members of the tic community often report that "artificial" or "synthetic" colors are triggers, without specifying a particular dye. More than one color is often used in a given product, making specific identification more difficult. It is a good practice to simply avoid all of them.

Approved dyes in the U.S.A. include the following list. (This approval does not apply to all countries.)

> FD&C Blue No. 1
> FD&C Blue No. 2
> FD&C Green No. 3
> FD&C Red No. 40
> FD&C Red No. 3
> FD&C Yellow No. 5
> FD&C Yellow No. 6
> Orange B (used in hot dog and sausage casings)

Also, note that brown caramel coloring, not included in this list, is sometimes made from sugar, but it can also be made from synthetic chemicals. Caramel coloring is often used in colas and other sodas, beer, brown bread, puddings, chocolates, and Chinese sauces. If you are not sure of the source, it is best to avoid it.

On the topic of artificial food dyes, the past-president of Center for Science in the Pubic Interest, Michael F. Jacobson, pointed out: "Major food companies like Coca-Cola, General Mills, McDonald's, and PepsiCo should be embarrassed that they are selling their American customers foods colored with Yellow 5, Yellow 6, Red 40, and other synthetic dyes, even as they are selling naturally colored or dye-free versions of the same foods in Europe.

American children will continue to be exposed to these powerful chemicals so long as the FDA lags behind its European counterparts."

Learn to read labels of foods and beverages. Avoid dyes, regardless of whether you have noticed an increase in tics or not. While it is not always possible to find medications without synthetic coloring, it can be worth the effort to look for dye-free versions. See *Feingold.org* for more information.

Flavorings

Many prepared foods have flavorings added. Those that do should specify the ingredient(s). Spices, herbs, and vanilla (not vanillin, which is synthetic) are examples of genuine natural flavorings. Unfortunately, the term "natural flavoring" as an added ingredient is widely used, and the item can contain synthetic flavorings. Each "flavor" can consist of hundreds of chemicals. They are often derived from petroleum, which is also the source for synthetic dyes and the three main preservatives BHA, BHT and TBHQ.

Flavorings are a complicated issue and can be explored online. The Feingold Association publishes lists of thousands of brand name products they have researched and are free of artificial flavorings, as well as synthetic dyes and the preservatives BHA, BHT, and TBHQ. Please refer to our *www.Latitudes. org/Trigger-Resources* pages for related web links.

MSG: Monosodium Glutamate

MSG is a flavor enhancer, processed from glutamic acid. Used in a wide range of food products, it is often associated with Chinese food but is included in many items like soups, salad dressings, snacks, seasoning salts, condiments and more. It is well known for being a potential headache trigger, and also for being disguised or hidden under different names. See pages 59-60 for more details. Not everyone is highly sensitive to this additive, but some have a significant negative reaction. See also: *www.MSGmyth.com*

Other foods additives to avoid

The Environmental Working Group singled out a number of preservatives and other additives that it recommends be avoided, in addition to flavorings and dye. Studies have suggested that each item below can be a hormone disruptor, a carcinogen, and/or detrimental to the nervous system. This is a partial list of items to watch for when reading labels.

- Nitrites and nitrates
- Potassium bromate
- Propyl paraben
- Butylated hydroxyanisole (BHA)
- Butylated hydroxytoluene (BHT)
- Propyl gallate
- Theobromine
- Diacetyl
- Phosphates
- Aluminum additives

Sweeteners

Over-consumption of sugar and high-fructose corn syrup is detrimental to health. Knowing this, millions of people turn to artificial sweeteners, but there are safety concerns with some of them. Aspartame is widely thought to be the most harmful, followed by acesulfame potassium (trade names Sunett and Sweet One in the USA, E950 in Europe); saccharin, and sucralose (Splenda). Stevia is considered one of the safest substitutes, especially an organic whole leaf stevia product and/or with no additional additives.

Appendix B: Salicylates and tyramine

Salicylates

A small percentage of people react to a group of naturally occurring chemicals known as salicylates. Salicylates are found in aspirin and certain other medications, select foods, and some products such as cosmetics. Responses can range from a mild to a serious allergic reaction. A large number of natural and typically healthful foods contain salicylates. Examples are almonds, apples, apricots, cherries, cranberries, cucumbers, grapes, oranges, nectarines, peaches, peppers, plums, prunes, raisins, tangerines, and tomatoes. If you suspect any of these may be troublesome for you, you may want to get a complete list and try avoiding foods with salicylates, monitoring to see if symptoms improve. A dietitian or allergist should be able to advise you on this topic. For helpful information on salicylates, search websites for the Feingold Association, Foods Matter, and Food Intolerance Network.

Tyramine

Tyramine occurs naturally in certain foods from a breakdown of the amino acid tyrosine. Some people are highly sensitive to it, and it is recognized as a trigger for migraine. Based on feedback to ACN (*Latitudes.org*), foods containing tyramine can also aggravate tics in some people who have a sensitivity to it. A summary of key foods containing high levels of tyramine includes, in part, meats, poultry or fish that are spoiled or pickled, fermented, smoked, aged, or marinated; and most pork and processed meats. Others are alcoholic beverages, aged cheeses, avocado*, banana*, chocolate, coconut, edamame, fava and other select beans, figs, kimchi, miso soup, peanuts, pecans, pineapple, plums, raspberries, sauerkraut, snow peas, sour cream, soy sauce, tempeh, teriyaki sauce, walnuts, yeast, and yogurt. See *Migraine.com* for a full list.

Especially when overripe

Appendix C: Migraine and headache triggers

As mentioned previously in this book, not everyone with a given condition experiences the same triggers, the same degree of response, nor the same number of triggers. The list of potential migraine and headache triggers that follows was obtained from *MayoClinic.com* and *National Institutes of Health* (NIH *and Medline Plus*) websites.

Many similarities can be seen between these migraine triggers and those on our tic trigger lists in Chapter 7. Although our lists related to tics are more detailed, these migraine and headache triggers gleaned from mainstream medical sources reinforce the validity of feedback that ACN (*Latitudes.org*) has received.

According to a research article by Zaeem (2016), the presence of any specific dietary trigger in migraine patients varies widely in the literature depending on the study population and methodology. It is noted that some foods trigger headache within an hour, while some symptoms tend to develop within 12 hours after eating.[44]

A *unique study on children, food, and headache*

Research published in March 2017 by Dr. S. Taheri examined common food triggers in a group of youngsters. He found that almost 90% of subjects eliminated their headaches during the study: "Effect of exclusion of frequently consumed dietary triggers in a cohort of children with chronic primary headache."

For this study, 115 children aged 3-15 years with primary headache were followed in a pediatric outpatient clinic. Patients who frequently consumed foods or food additives generally known to trigger headaches were advised to exclude those items, two at a time, for six weeks and return for follow-up with a headache and food diary. Reportedly, 87% of the participants achieved "complete resolution of headaches" by exclusion of 1 to 3 of the identified food(s). Thirteen percent did not respond to the food exclusion.

The most frequent food triggers the children experienced were, in order of frequency: 1) Caffeine; 2) monosodium glutamate (MSG); 3) cocoa; 4) aspartame; 5) cheese; 6) citrus; 7) and nitrites.

The study concluded "This is the first study to show that headaches can be triggered by the *cumulative effect of a food that is frequently consumed*, rather than by a single time ingestion."[45]

Migraine headache triggers

- Aged cheeses
- Alcohol
- Anxiety
- Aspartame
- Baked goods
- Bright and flashing lights/sun glare
- Caffeinated beverages
- Chicken livers
- Chocolate
- Dairy foods, especially cheese
- Dehydration
- Emotional stress
- Foods with tyramine (see p. 168)
- Fruits (avocado, banana, citrus)
- Hormonal changes
- Loud sounds
- Meats containing nitrates
- Medications: oral contraceptives and vasodilators

- MSG (monosodium glutamate)
- Onions
- Peanuts and other nuts/seeds
- Processed, fermented, pickled, or marinated foods
- Red wine
- Salty foods
- Sensory issues
- Skipping meals or fasting
- Smell of paint thinner
- Smell of perfume
- Smoked fish
- Stress

Also
- Intense physical exertion
- Changes in wake-sleep patterns
- Change in weather/barometric pressure

Sources: MayoClinic.com and National Institutes of Health (NIH and Medline Plus)

Notes

Numbered text references

1. Okun, Michael S. *Tourette Syndrome: 10 Secrets to a Happier Life.* Books4Patients, March 1, 2017.

2. Mathews, Carol A., and Jeremy S. Stern. "The First World Congress on Tourette Syndrome and Tic Disorders: Controversies and Hot Topics in Etiology and Treatment." *Frontiers in Neuroscience* 10 (2016).

3. American Psychiatric Association. *Diagnostic and Statistical Manual of Mental Disorders: DSM-5.* 2013.

4. Black, Kevin J., Elizabeth R. Black, Deanna J. Greene, and Bradley L. Schlaggar. "Provisional Tic Disorder: What to Tell Parents When their Child First Starts Ticcing." F1000 *Research* 5 (2016), 696.

5. Robertson, Mary M. "A personal 35 year perspective on Gilles de la Tourette syndrome: prevalence, phenomenology, comorbidities, and coexistent psycho-pathologies." *The Lancet Psychiatry* 2, no. 1 (2015), 68-87.

6. Kurlan, R., M. P. McDermott, C. Deeley, P. G. Como, C. Brower, S. Eapen, E. M. Andresen, and B. Miller. "Prevalence of Tics in Schoolchildren and Association with Placement in Special Education." *Neurology* 57, no. 8 (2001), 1383-1388.

7. Pappert, E. J., C. G. Goetz, E. D. Louis, L. Blasucci, and S. Leurgans. "Objective Assessments of Longitudinal Outcome in Gilles de la Tourette's Syndrome." *Neurology* 61, no. 7 (2003), 936-940.

8. Hirschtritt, Matthew E., Paul C. Lee, David L. Pauls, Yves Dion, Marco A. Grados, Cornelia Illmann, Robert A. King, et al. "Lifetime Prevalence, Age of Risk, and Genetic Relationships of Comorbid Psychiatric Disorders in Tourette Syndrome." JAMA *Psychiatry* 72, no. 4 (2015), 325.

9. Roessner, Veit, Kerstin J. Plessen, Aribert Rothenberger, Andrea G. Ludolph, Renata Rizzo, Liselotte Skov, et al. "European Clinical Guidelines for Tourette Syndrome and other Tic Disorders. Part II: Pharmacological Treatment." *European Child & Adolescent Psychiatry* 20, no. 4 (2011), 173-196.

10. Zhang, Jian-Guo, Yan Ge, Matt Stead, Kai Zhang, Shuang-shuang Yan, Wei Hu, and Fan-Gang Meng. "Long-term Outcome of Globus Pallidus Internus Deep Brain Stimulation in Patients With Tourette Syndrome." *Mayo Clinic Proceedings* 89, no. 11 (2014), 1506-1514.

11. Scahill, Lawrence, Douglas W. Woods, Michael B. Himle, Alan L. Peterson, Sabine Wilhelm, John C. Piacentini, Kevin McNaught, John T. Walkup, and Jonathan

W. Mink. "Current Controversies on the Role of Behavior therapy in Tourette Syndrome." *Movement Disorders* 28, no. 9 (2013), 1179-1183.

12. DeMare, Sheila Rogers *Natural Treatments for Tics & Tourette's: A Patient and Family Guide.* Berkeley, Calif: North Atlantic Books, 2008.

13. Chao, Ting-Kuang, Jing Hu, and Tamara Pringsheim. "Prenatal Risk Factors for Tourette Syndrome: A Systematic Review." *BMC Pregnancy and Childbirth* 14, no. 1 (2014).

14. Brauser, D. "Potential New Risk Factors for Tourette's, Tics Identified." *Medscape.* Accessed June 20, 2017. http://www.medscape.com/viewarticle/819287.

15. Mataix-Cols, David, Kayoko Isomura, Ana Pérez-Vigil, Zheng Chang, Christian Rück, K. J. Larsson, James F. Leckman, et al. "Familial Risks of Tourette Syndrome and Chronic Tic Disorders." *JAMA Psychiatry* 72, no. 8 (2015), 787.

16. Mathews, C. A., J. M. Scharf, L. L. Miller, C. Macdonald-Wallis, D. A. Lawlor, and Y. Ben-Shlomo. "Association between Pre- and Perinatal Exposures and Tourette Syndrome or Chronic Tic Disorder in the ALSPAC Cohort." *The British Journal of Psychiatry* 204, no. 1 (2013), 40-45.

17. Ghosh, Debabrata, Prashant V. Rajan, Deepanjana Das, Priya Datta, A. D. Rothner, and Gerald Erenberg. "Headache in Children with Tourette Syndrome." *The Journal of Pediatrics* 161, no. 2 (2012), 303-307.

18. Silva-Néto, RP, MFP Peres, and MM Valença. "Odorant Substances that Trigger Headaches in Migraine Patients." *Cephalalgia* 34, no. 1 (2014), 14-21.

19. Fornazieri, Marco A., Anibal R. Neto, Fabio De Rezende Pinna, Fabio H. Gobbi Porto, Paulo De Lima Navarro, Richard L. Voegels, and Richard L. Doty. "Olfactory Symptoms Reported by Migraineurs With and Without Auras." *Headache: The Journal of Head and Face Pain* 56, no. 10 (2016), 1608-1616.

20. Perlmutter, David, and Carol Colman. *The Better Brain Book: The Best Tools for Improving Memory, Sharpness, and Preventing Aging of the Brain.* New York: Riverhead Books, 2005.

21. Gehle, Kimberly S., Jewel L. Crawford, and Michael T. Hatcher. "Integrating Environmental Health Into Medical Education." *American Journal of Preventive Medicine* 41, no. 4 (2011), S296-S301.

22. Schenk, M., S. M. Popp, A. V. Neale, and R. Y. Demers. "Environmental Medicine Content in Medical School Curricula." *Academic Medicine* 71, no. 5 (1996), 499-501.

23. Galland, Leo, and Jonathan Galland. *The Allergy Solution: Unlock the Surprising, Hidden Truth About Why You Are Sick and How to Get Well.* Hay House, Inc. 2016.

24. Yuce, M., S. N. Guner, K. Karabekiroglu, et al. "Association of Tourette Syndrome and Obsessive-Compulsive Disorder with Allergic Diseases in Children and Adolescents: A Preliminary Study." *European Review for Medical and Pharmacological Sciences* 18, no. 3 (2014), 303-310.

25. Cacabelos, Ramón, Clara Torrellas, Lucía Fernández-Novoa, and Gjumrakch Aliev. "Neuroimmune Crosstalk in CNS Disorders: The Histamine Connection." *Current Pharmaceutical Design* 22, no. 7 (2016), 819-848.

26. Ho, C. S., Ein-Yiao Shen, Shyh-Dar Shyur, and Noah Chiu. "Association of Allergy with Tourette's Syndrome." *Journal of the Formosan Medical Association* 98, no. 7 (1999), 492-495.

27. Chang, Yu-Tzu, Yu-Fen Li, Chih-Hsin Muo, Shih-Chieh Chen, Zheng-Nan Chin, et al, "Correlation of Tourette Syndrome and Allergic Disease: Nationwide Population-Based Base-Control Study." *Journal of Developmental & Behavioral Pediatrics* 32, no. 2 (2011), 98-102.

28. Gerrard, John W., J. S. Richardson, and Jeffrey Donat. "Neuropharmacological Evaluation of Movement Disorders that are Adverse Reactions to Specific Foods." *International Journal of Neuroscience* 76, no. 1-2 (1994), 61-69.

29. Martin, Vincent T., and Brinder Vij. "Diet and Headache: Part 1." *Headache: The Journal of Head and Face Pain* 56, no. 9 (2016), 1543-1552.

30. Verstraten, T., Davis RL, DeStefano F, Lieu TA, Rhodes PH, Black SB, Shinefield H, Chen RT; Vaccine Safety Datalink Team. Safety of thimerosal-containing vaccines: a two-phased study of computerized health maintenance organization databases. *Pediatrics.* 2003 Nov;112(5):1039-48.

31. Andrews, N. "Thimerosal Exposure in Infants and Developmental Disorders: A Retrospective Cohort Study in the United Kingdom Does Not Support a Causal Association." *Pediatrics* 114, no. 3 (2004), 584-591. ***Note from Sheila Rogers DeMare:** Regardless of the article title, the journal text states that no association was found "with the possible exception of tics."

32. Young, Heather A., David A. Geier, and Mark R. Geier. "Thimerosal exposure in infants and neurodevelopmental disorders: An assessment of computerized medical records in the Vaccine Safety Datalink." *Journal of the Neurological Sciences* 271, no. 1-2 (2008), 110-118.

33. Geier, David A., and Mark R. Geier. "Neurodevelopmental Disorders Following Thimerosal-Containing Childhood Immunizations: A Follow-Up Analysis." *International Journal of Toxicology* 23, no. 6 (2004),

34. Leslie, Douglas L., Robert A. Kobre, Brian J. Richmand, Selin Aktan Guloksuz, and James F. Leckman. "Temporal Association of Certain Neuropsychiatric Disorders Following Vaccination of Children and Adolescents: A Pilot Case–Control Study." *Frontiers in Psychiatry* 8 (2017).

35. Steinemann, Anne. "Health and societal effects from exposure to fragranced consumer products." *Preventive Medicine Reports* 5 (2017), 45-47.

36. Russo, Antonio, Antonio Bruno, Francesca Trojsi, Alessandro Tessitore, and Gioacchino Tedeschi. "Lifestyle Factors and Migraine in Childhood." *Current Pain and Headache Reports* 20, no. 2 (2016).

37. Silva-Néto, RP, MFP Peres, and MM Valença. "Odorant Substances that Trigger Headaches in Migraine Patients." *Cephalalgia* 34, no. 1 (2014), 14-21.

38. Ashford, Nicholas Askounes, and Claudia Miller. *Chemical Exposures: Low Levels and High Stakes.* New York: Van Nostrand Reinhold, 1997.

39. Miller, Claudia S. "The Compelling Anomaly of Chemical Intolerance." *Annals of the New York Academy of Sciences* 933, no. 1 (2006), 1-23.

40. Radetsky, Peter. *Allergic to the Twentieth Century: The Explosion in Environmental Allergies - from Sick Buildings to Multiple Chemical Sensitivity.* Boston: Little, Brown, 1997

41. Dunckley, Victoria L. *Reset Your Child's Brain: A Four-Week Plan to End Meltdowns, Raise Grades, and Boost Social Skills by Reversing the Effects of Electronic Screen-Time.* New World Library, Novato, CA, 2015.

42. Wigle, D. T. *Child Health and the Environment.* New York: Oxford University Press, 2003.

43. Chang, Kiki, Jennifer Frankovich, Michael Cooperstock, Madeleine W. Cunningham, M. E. Latimer, Tanya K. Murphy, Mark Pasternack, et al. "Clinical Evaluation of Youth with Pediatric Acute-Onset Neuropsychiatric Syndrome (PANS): Recommendations from the 2013 PANS Consensus Conference." *Journal of Child and Adolescent Psychopharmacology* 25, no. 1 (2015), 3-13.

44. Zaeem, Zoya, Lily Zhou, and Esma Dilli. "Headaches: a Review of the Role of Dietary Factors." *Current Neurology and Neuroscience Reports* 16, no. 11 (2016).

45. Taheri, Sepideh. "Effect of exclusion of frequently consumed dietary triggers in a cohort of children with chronic primary headache." *Nutrition and Health* 23, no. 1 (2017), 47-50.

Additional Reading

On tics and Tourette syndrome

1. Altindag, Abdurrahman, Medaim Yanik, and Mehmet Asoglu. "The emergence of tics during escitalopram and sertraline treatment." *International Clinical Psychopharmacology* 20, no. 3 (2005), 177-178.

2. Alves, Helvio L., and Elizabeth M. Quagliato. "The Prevalence of Tic Disorders in Children and Adolescents in Brazil." *Arquivos de Neuro-Psiquiatria* 72, no. 12 (2014), 942-948.

3. Capuano, Alessandro, and Giovanni Valeri. "Tics and Tourette Syndrome in Autism Spectrum Disorder." *Psychiatric Symptoms and Comorbidities in Autism Spectrum Disorder*, 2016, 93-109.

4. Castellan Baldan, Lissandra, Kyle A. Williams, Jean-Dominique Gallezot, Vladimir Pogorelov, Maximiliano Rapanelli, Michael Crowley, George M. Anderson, et al. "Histidine Decarboxylase Deficiency Causes Tourette Syndrome: Parallel Findings in Humans and Mice." *Neuron* 81, no. 1 (2014), 77-90.

5. Caurín, Belén, Mercedes Serrano, Emilio Fernández-Alvarez, Jaume Campistol, and Belén Pérez-Dueñas. "Environmental circumstances influencing tic expression in children." *European Journal of Paediatric Neurology* 18, no. 2 (2014), 157-162.

6. "Diagnosing Tic Disorders." Tourette Syndrome | NCBDDD | CDC. Accessed April 19, 2017. https://www.cdc.gov/ncbddd/tourette/diagnosis.html.

7. Forde, Natalie J., Ahmad S. Kanaan, Joanna Widomska, Shanmukha S. Padmanabhuni, Ester Nespoli, John Alexander, Juan I. Rodriguez Arranz, et al. "TS-EUROTRAIN: A European-Wide Investigation and Training Network on the Etiology and Pathophysiology of Gilles de la Tourette Syndrome." *Frontiers in Neuroscience* 10 (2016).

8. Fredericksen, K.A., L.E. Cutting, W.R. Kates, S.H. Mostofsky, H.S. Singer, K.L. Cooper, D.C. Lanham, M.B. Denckla, and W.E. Kaufmann. "Disproportionate Increases of White Matter in Right Frontal Lobe in Tourette Syndrome." *Neurology* 58, no. 1 (2002), 85-89.

9. Freeman, Roger D., Diane K. Fast, Larry Burd, Jacob Kerbeshian, Mary M. Robertson, and Paul Sandor. "An International Perspective on Tourette Syndrome: Selected Findings from 3500 Individuals in 22 countries." *Developmental Medicine & Child Neurology* 42, no. 7 (2000), 436-447.

10. Frick, Luciana, and Christopher Pittenger. "Microglial Dysregulation in OCD,

Tourette Syndrome, and PANDAS." *Journal of Immunology Research* (2016), 1-8.

11. Harding, G.F.A., and P.F. Harding. "Photosensitive Epilepsy and Image Safety." *Applied Ergonomics* 41, no. 4 (2010), 504-508.

12. Hauser, Robert A., and Theresa A. Zesiewicz. "Sertraline-induced exacerbation of Tics in Tourette's syndrome." *Movement Disorders* 10, no. 5 (1995), 682-684.

13. Hoekstra, Pieter J., Andrea Dietrich, Mark J. Edwards, Ishraga Elamin, and Davide Martino. "Environmental Factors in Tourette Syndrome." *Neuroscience & Biobehavioral Reviews* 37, no. 6 (2013), 1040-1049.

14. Hyde, T. M. "Tourette's syndrome. A model neuropsychiatric disorder." JAMA: *The Journal of the American Medical Association* 273, no. 6 (1995), 498-501.

15. Khalifa, Najah, and Anne-Liis Von Knorring. "Prevalence of tic disorders and Tourette syndrome in a Swedish school population." *Developmental Medicine & Child Neurology* 45, no. 05 (2003).

16. Kawikova, Ivana, Bart P. Grady, Zuzana Tobiasova, Yan Zhang, Aristo Vojdani, Liliya Katsovich, Brian J. Richmand, Tae W. Park, Alfred L. Bothwell, and James F. Leckman. "Children with Tourette's Syndrome May Suffer Immunoglobulin A Dysgammaglobulinemia: Preliminary Report." *Biological Psychiatry* 67, no. 7 (2010), 679-683.

17. Mantel, Barbara J., Andrea Meyers, Quan Y. Tran, Sheila Rogers, and Judith S. Jacobson. "Nutritional Supplements and Complementary/Alternative Medicine in Tourette Syndrome." *Journal of Child and Adolescent Psychopharmacology* 14, no. 4 (2004), 582-589.

18. Mathews, Carol A., and Marco A. Grados. "Familiality of Tourette Syndrome, Obsessive-Compulsive Disorder, and Attention-Deficit/Hyperactivity Disorder: Heritability Analysis in a Large Sib-Pair Sample." *Journal of the American Academy of Child & Adolescent Psychiatry* 50, no. 1 (2011), 46-54.

19. Kompoliti, Katie, Wenqin Fan, and Sue Leurgans. "Complementary and alternative medicine use in Gilles de la Tourette syndrome." *Movement Disorders* 24, no. 13 (2009), 2015-2019.

20. Leckman, James F. "Tourette's syndrome." *The Lancet* 360, no. 9345 (2002), 1577-1586.

21. Leckman, J. F., H. Zhang, A. Vitale, F. Lahnin, K. Lynch, C. Bondi, Y.-S. Kim, and B. S. Peterson. "Course of tic severity in Tourette syndrome: The first two decades." *Pediatrics* 102, no. 1 (1998), 14-19.

22. Li, Erzhen, Yiyan Ruan, Qian Chen, Xiaodai Cui, Lingyun Lv, Ping Zheng, and Liwen Wang. "Streptococcal infection and immune response in children with Tourette's syndrome." *Child's Nervous System* 31, no. 7 (2015), 1157-1163.

23. Lit, Lisa, Amanda Enstrom, Frank R. Sharp, and Donald L. Gilbert. "Age-related gene expression in Tourette syndrome." *Journal of Psychiatric Research* 43, no. 3 (2009), 319-330.

24. Jankovic, Joseph, and Roger Kurlan. "Tourette syndrome: Evolving concepts." *Movement Disorders* 26, no. 6 (2011), 1149-1156.

25. Martino, Davide, Panagiotis Zis, and Maura Buttiglione. "The role of immune mechanisms in Tourette syndrome." *Brain Research* 1617 (2015), 126-143.

26. McGuire, Joseph F., John Piacentini, Erin A. Brennan, Adam B. Lewin, Tanya K. Murphy, Brent J. Small, and Eric A. Storch. "A Meta-Analysis of Behavior Therapy for Tourette Syndrome." *Journal of Psychiatric Research* 50 (2014), 106-112.

27. Mink, Jonathan W., John Walkup, Kirk A. Frey, Peter Como, Danielle Cath, Mahlon R. DeLong, Gerald Erenberg, et al. "Patient Selection and Assessment Recommendations for Deep Brain Stimulation in Tourette Syndrome." *Movement Disorders* 21, no. 11 (2006), 1831-1838.

28. Motlagh, Maria G., Liliya Katsovich, Nancy Thompson, Haiqun Lin, Young-Shin Kim, Lawrence Scahill, et al, "Severe Psychosocial Stress and Heavy Cigarette Smoking During Pregnancy: An Examination of the Pre- and Perinatal Risk Factors Associated with ADHD and Tourette Syndrome." *European Child & Adolescent Psychiatry* 19, no. 10 (2010), 755-764.

29. Müller-Vahl, Kirsten R., Nadine Buddensiek, Menedimos Geomelas, and Hinderk M. Emrich. "The Influence of Different Food and Drink on Tics in Tourette Syndrome." *Acta Paediatrica* 97, no. 4 (2008), 442-446.

30. Muellner, Julia, Christine Delmaire, Romain Valabrégue, Michael Schüpbach, Jean-François Mangin, Marie Vidailhet, et al. "Altered Structure of Cortical Sulci in Gilles de la Tourette Syndrome: Further Support for Abnormal Brain Development." *Movement Disorders* 30, no. 5 (2015), 655-661.

31. Murphy, Tanya K., Roger Kurlan, and James Leckman. "The Immunobiology of Tourette's Disorder, Pediatric Autoimmune Neuropsychiatric Disorders Associated with Streptococcus , and Related Disorders: A Way Forward." *Journal of Child and Adolescent Psychopharmacology* 20, no. 4 (2010), 317-331.

32. Pagliaroli, Luca, Borbála Vető, Tamás Arányi, and Csaba Barta. "From Genetics to Epigenetics: New Perspectives in Tourette Syndrome Research." *Frontiers in*

Neuroscience 10 (2016).

33. Plessen, Kerstin J., Ravi Bansal, and Bradley S. Peterson. "Imaging Evidence for Anatomical Disturbances and Neuroplastic Compensation in Persons with Tourette Syndrome." *Journal of Psychosomatic Research* 67, no. 6 (2009), 559-573.

34. Pourfar, M., A. Feigin, C. C. Tang, M. Carbon-Correll, M. Bussa, C. Budman, V. Dhawan, and D. Eidelberg. "Abnormal Metabolic Brain Networks in Tourette Syndrome." *Neurology* 76, no. 11 (2011), 944-952.

35. Rapp, Doris J. *Is This Your Child?: Discovering and Treating Unrecognized Allergies.* New York: W. Morrow, 1991.

36. Robertson, Mary M. "A Personal 35 Year Perspective on Gilles de la Tourette Syndrome: Prevalence, Phenomenology, Comorbidities, and Coexistent Psychopathologies." *The Lancet Psychiatry* 2, no. 1 (2015), 68-87.

37. Robertson, Mary M. "The Gilles De La Tourette syndrome: the current status." Archives of disease in childhood - *Education & Practice* edition 97, no. 5 (2012), 166-175.

38. Robertson, Mary M. "The prevalence and epidemiology of Gilles de la Tourette syndrome." *Journal of Psychosomatic Research* 65, no. 5 (2008), 461-472.

39. Scharf, Jeremiah M., Laura L. Miller, Caitlin A. Gauvin, Janelle Alabiso, Carol A. Mathews, and Yoav Ben-Shlomo. "Population Prevalence of Tourette Syndrome: A Systematic Review and Meta-Analysis." *Movement Disorders* 30, no. 2 (2014), 221-228.

40. Snider, L. A., L. D. Seligman, B. R. Ketchen, S. J. Levitt, L. R. Bates, M. A. Garvey, and S. E. Swedo. "Tics and Problem Behaviors in Schoolchildren: Prevalence, Characterization, and Associations." *Pediatrics* 110, no. 2 (2002), 331-336.

41. Silva, Raul R., Dinohra M. Munoz, Julia Barickman, and Arnold J. Friedhoff. "Environmental Factors and Related Fluctuation of Symptoms in Children and Adolescents with Tourette's Disorder." *Journal of Child Psychology and Psychiatry* 36, no. 2 (1995), 305-312.

42. Spinello, Chiara, Giovanni Laviola, and Simone Macrì. "Pediatric Autoimmune Disorders Associated with Streptococcal Infections and Tourette's Syndrome in Preclinical Studies." *Frontiers in Neuroscience* 10 (2016).

43. Swain, James E., Lawrence Scahill, Paul J Lombroso, Robert A King, and James F. Leckman. "Tourette Syndrome and Tic Disorders: A Decade of Progress." *Journal of the American Academy of Child & Adolescent Psychiatry* 46, no. 8 (2007), 947-968.

44. Tsai, Ching-Shu, Yao-Hsu Yang, Kuo-You Huang, Yena Lee, Roger S. McIntyre, and Vincent C. Chen. "Association of Tic Disorders and Enterovirus Infection."

Medicine 95, no. 15 (2016), e3347.

45. Yang, Jaeun, Lauren Hirsch, Davide Martino, Nathalie Jette, Jodie Roberts, and Tamara Pringsheim. "The Prevalence of Diagnosed Tourette Syndrome in Canada: A national Population-Based Study." *Movement Disorders* 31, no. 11 (2016), 1658-1663.

46. Yeh, Chin-Bin, Ching-Hsing Wu, Hui-Chu Tsung, Chia-Wei Chen, Jia-Fwu Shyu, and James F. Leckman. "Antineural Antibody in Patients with Tourette's Syndrome and their Family Members." *Journal of Biomedical Science* 13, no. 1 (2005), 101-112.41.

47. Zilhão, N. R., M. C. Olthof, D. J. Smit, D. C. Cath, L. Ligthart, C. A. Mathews, K. Delucchi, D. I. Boomsma, and C. V. Dolan. "Heritability of tic disorders: a twin-family study." *Psychological Medicine* 47, no. 06 (2016), 1085-1096.

48. Zilhão, Nuno R., Shanmukha S. Padmanabhuni, Luca Pagliaroli, Csaba Barta, Dirk J. Smit, Danielle Cath, Michel G. Nivard, et al. "Epigenome-Wide Association Study of Tic Disorders." *Twin Research and Human Genetics* 18, no. 06 (2015), 699-709.

49. Zou, Li-Ping, Ying Wang, Li-Ping Zhang, Jian-Bo Zhao, Jin-Fang Lu, Qun Liu, and Hang-Yan Wang. "Tourette syndrome and excitatory substances: is there a connection?" *Child's Nervous System* 27, no. 5 (2010), 793-802.

On environmental and allergic issues: non-specific

1. Brostoff, Jonathan, and Linda Gamlin. *Food Allergies and Food Intolerance: The Complete Guide to Their Identification and Treatment.* Rochester, Vt: Healing Arts Press, 2000.

2. Chad, Zave. "Allergies in Children." *Paediatrics & Child Health* 6, no. 8 (2001), 555-566.

3. Farmer, S. A., T. D. Nelin, M. J. Falvo, and L. E. Wold. "Ambient and household air pollution: complex triggers of disease." AJP: *Heart and Circulatory Physiology* 307, no. 4 (2014), H467-H476.

4. Goldberg, Aaron D., C. D. Allis, and Emily Bernstein. "Epigenetics: A landscape takes shape." *Cell* 128, no. 4 (2007), 635-638.

5. Miller, Claudia, Nicholas Ashford, Richard Doty, Mary Lamielle, David Otto, Alice Rahill, and Lance Wallace. "Empirical Approaches for the Investigation of Toxicant-Induced Loss of Tolerance." *Environmental Health Perspectives* 105 (1997), 515.

6. Roberts, John W., Lance A. Wallace, David E. Camann, Philip Dickey, Steven G. Gilbert, Robert G. Lewis, and Tim K. Takaro. "Monitoring and Reducing Exposure of Infants to Pollutants in House Dust." *Reviews of Environmental Contamination and Toxicology* Vol 201, 2009, 1-39.

7. Philpott, William H., and Dwight K. Kalita. *Brain Allergies: The Psycho-Nutrient Connection.* New Canaan, Conn: Keats Pub, 1980.

8. Rapp, Doris J. *Our Toxic World, a Wake Up Call: How to Keep Yourself and Your Loved Ones Out of Harm's Way: Chemicals Damage Your Body, Brain, Behavior and Sex.* Buffalo, N.Y.: Environmental Medical Research Foundation, 2004.

9. Sicherer, Scott H. "IgE- and Non-IgE-Mediated Food Allergy." *Eosinophilic Esophagitis*, 2011, 219-238.

10. Vojdani, Aristo. "Molecular mimicry as a mechanism for food immune reactivities and autoimmunity." *Alternative Therapies in Health and Medicine*, Supplement 1, 21 (2015), 34-45.

11. Yuede, Carla, John Olney, and Catherine Creeley. "Developmental Neurotoxicity of Alcohol and Anesthetic Drugs Is Augmented by Co-Exposure to Caffeine." *Brain Sciences* 3, no. 3 (2013), 1128-1152.

On triggers for medical conditions including ADHD

1. Alicea-Alvarez, Norma, Foppiano Palacios, Melanie Ortiz, Diana Huang, and Kathleen Reeves. "Path to health asthma study: A survey of pediatric asthma in an urban community." *Journal of Asthma*, 54, no.3 (2016), 273-278.

2. Ananthakrishnan, Ashwin N. "Environmental Risk Factors for Inflammatory Bowel Diseases: A Review." *Digestive Diseases and Sciences* 60, no. 2 (2015), 290-298.

3. Atan Sahin, Ozlem, Nuray Kececioglu, Muhittin Serdar, and Aysel Ozpinar. "The association of residential mold exposure and adenotonsillar hypertrophy in children living in damp environments." *International Journal of Pediatric Otorhinolaryngology* 88 (2016), 233-238.

4. Arnold, L. E., Nicholas Lofthouse, and Elizabeth Hurt. "Artificial Food Colors and Attention-Deficit/Hyperactivity Symptoms: Conclusions to Dye for." *Neurotherapeutics* 9, no. 3 (2012), 599-609.

5. Barichella, Michela, Emanuele Cereda, Erica Cassani, Giovanna Pinelli, Laura Iorio, Valentina Ferri, Giulia Privitera, et al. "Dietary habits and neurological features of Parkinson's disease patients: Implications for practice." *Clinical Nutrition*, 36, no.4 (2017), 1054-1061.

6. Bektas, Hesna, Hayriye Karabulut, Beyza Doganay, and Baran Acar. "Allergens might trigger migraine attacks." *Acta Neurologica Belgica* 117, no. 1 (2016), 91-95.

7. Bolton, D. J., and L. J. Robertson. "Mental Health Disorders Associated with Foodborne Pathogens." *Journal of Food Protection* 79, no. 11 (2016), 2005-2017.

8. Chansky, Tamar E. *Freeing Yourself from Anxiety: Four Simple Steps to Overcome Worry and Create the Life You Want.* Cambridge, MA: Da Capo Life Long, 2012.

9. Demarquay, Geneviève, and François Mauguière. "Central Nervous System Underpinnings of Sensory Hypersensitivity in Migraine: Insights from Neuroimaging and Electrophysiological Studies." *Headache: The Journal of Head and Face Pain* 56, no. 9 (2015), 1418-1438.

10. Faber, Scott, Gregory M. Zinn, Andrew Boggess, Timothy Fahrenholz, John C. Kern, and HM S. Kingston. "A cleanroom sleeping environment's impact on markers of oxidative stress, immune dysregulation, and behavior in children with autism spectrum disorders." BMC *Complementary and Alternative Medicine* 15, no. 1 (2015).

11. Fogel, O., C. Richard-Miceli, and J. Tost. "Epigenetic Changes in Chronic Inflammatory Diseases." *Advances in Protein Chemistry and Structural Biology,* (2017), 139-189.

12. Ghalichi, Faezeh, Jamal Ghaemmaghami, Ayyoub Malek, and Alireza Ostadrahimi. "Effect of gluten free diet on gastrointestinal and behavioral indices for children with autism spectrum disorders: a randomized clinical trial." *World Journal of Pediatrics* 12, no. 4 (2016), 436-442.

13. Greenblatt, James, "Integrative Therapies for the Treatment of ADHD," Great Plains video. 1:01, April 5, 2013 https://vimeo.com/63408550.

14. Greenblatt, James, and Bill Gottlieb. *Finally Focused: The Breakthrough Natural Treatment Plan for Adhd That Restores Attention, Minimizes Hyperactivity, and Helps Eliminate Drug Side Effects.* 2017.

15. Gulati, Gaurav, and Hermine I. Brunner. "Environmental triggers in systemic lupus erythematosus." Seminars in Arthritis and Rheumatism, 2017.

16. Heilskov Rytter, Maren Joanne, Louise Beltroft Borup Andersen, Tine Houmann, Niels Bilenberg, Allan Hvolby, Christian Mølgaard, et al. "Diet in the treatment of ADHD in children—A systematic review of the literature." *Nordic Journal of Psychiatry* 69, no. 1 (2014), 1-18.

17. Hersey, Jane. *Why Can't My Child Behave? Why Can't She Cope? Why Can't He Learn?* Pear Tree Press, 2014.

18. Jiao, Juan, Ann Vincent, Stephen S. Cha, Connie A. Luedtke, Chul H. Kim, and Terry H. Oh. "Physical Trauma and Infection as Precipitating Factors in Patients with Fibromyalgia." American Journal of Physical Medicine & Rehabilitation 94, no. 12 (2015)

19. Kalkbrenner, Amy E., Rebecca J. Schmidt, and Annie C. Penlesky. "Environmental Chemical Exposures and Autism Spectrum Disorders: A Review of the Epidemiological Evidence." Current Problems in Pediatric and Adolescent Health Care 44, no. 10 (2014), 277-318.

20. Kim, Stephani, Monica Arora, Cristina Fernandez, Julio Landero, Joseph Caruso, and Aimin Chen. "Lead, Mercury, and Cadmium Exposure and Attention Deficit Hyperactivity Disorder in Children." Environmental Research 126 (2013), 105-110.

21. Louis, Elan D. "Environmental Epidemiology of Essential Tremor." Neuro-epidemiology 31, no. 3 (2008), 139-149.

22. Louis, Elan D., Garrett A. Keating, Kenneth T. Bogen, Eileen Rios, Kathryn M. Pellegrino, and Pam Factor-Litvak. "Dietary Epidemiology of Essential Tremor: Meat Consumption and Meat Cooking Practices." Neuroepidemiology 30, no. 3 (2008), 161-166.

23. Louis, Elan D., Eva C. Jurewicz, and Michael K. Parides. "Case-Control Study of Nutritional Antioxidant Intake in Essential Tremor." Neuroepidemiology 24, no. 4 (2005), 203-208.

24. Mao, Weian. "Atopic Eczema: A Disease Modulated by Gene and Environment." Frontiers in Bioscience 19, no. 4 (2014), 707.

25. McCann, Donna, Angelina Barrett, Alison Cooper, Debbie Crumpler, Lindy Dalen, Kate Grimshaw, Elizabeth Kitchin, et al. "Food additives and hyperactive behaviour in 3-year-old and 8/9-year-old children in the community: a randomised, double-blinded, placebo-controlled trial." The Lancet 370, no. 9598 (2007), 1560-1567.

26. Millichap, J. G. "Video Game-Induced Seizures." Pediatric Neurology Briefs 8, no. 9 (1994), 68.

27. Moien-Afshari, Farzad, and José F. Téllez-Zenteno. "Occipital Seizures Induced by Hyperglycemia: A Case Report and Review of Literature." Seizure 18, no. 5 (2009), 382-385.

28. Myatt, Theodore, Taeko Minegishi, and David MacIntosh. "Asthma Triggers in Indoor Air." Environmental Health, 2013, 107-130.

29. Nielsen, Philip R., Tue W. Kragstrup, Bent W. Deleuran, and Michael E. Benros. "Infections as Risk Factor for Autoimmune Diseases–A Nationwide Study." Journal of Autoimmunity 74 (2016), 176-181.

30. Pelsser, Lidy M., Jan K. Buitelaar, and Huub F. Savelkoul. "ADHD as a (Non) Allergic Hypersensitivity Disorder: A Hypothesis." *Pediatric Allergy and Immunology* 20, no. 2 (2009), 107-112.

31. Peña, Amado S., and Luis Rodrigo. "Celiac Disease and Non-Celiac Gluten Sensitivity." *Celiac Disease and Non-Celiac Gluten Sensitivity*, 2014, 25-44.

32. Rist, Pamela M., Julie Buring, and Tobias Kurth. "Dietary patterns according to headache and migraine status." *Cephalalgia* 35, no. 9 (2015), 767-775.

33. Singh, Vijendra K., Sheren X. Lin, Elizabeth Newell, and Courtney Nelson. "Abnormal Measles-Mumps-Rubella Antibodies and CNS Autoimmunity in Children with Autism." *Journal of Biomedical Science* 9, no. 4 (2002), 359-364.

34. Steinemann, Anne. "Ten questions concerning air fresheners and indoor built environments." *Building and Environment* 111 (2017), 279-284.

35. Stevens, L. J., T. Kuczek, J. R. Burgess, E. Hurt, and L. E. Arnold. "Dietary Sensitivities and ADHD Symptoms: Thirty-five Years of Research." *Clinical Pediatrics* 50, no. 4 (2010), 279-293.

36. Timmermans, E.J., S. Van der Pas, L.A. Schaap, and D.J.H. Deeg. "Self-Perceived Weather Sensitivity and Joint Pain in Older People with Osteoarthritis in Six European Countries: Results from the European Project on OsteoArthritis (EPOSA)." *European Geriatric Medicine* 4 (2013), S24.

37. Van der Mark, Marianne, Roel Vermeulen, Peter C. Nijssen, Wim M. Mulleners, Antonetta M. Sas, Teus Van Laar, et al. "Occupational Exposure to Pesticides and Endotoxin and Parkinson Disease in the Netherlands." *Occupational and Environmental Medicine* 71, no. 11 (2014), 757-764.

38. Van der Schans, Jurjen, Janine C. Pleiter, Tjalling W. De Vries, Catharina C. Schuiling-Veninga, Jens H. Bos, Pieter J. Hoekstra, and Eelko Hak. "Association between Medication Prescription for Atopic Diseases and Attention-Deficit/Hyperactivity Disorder." *Annals of Allergy, Asthma & Immunology* 117, no. 2 (2016), 186-191.

39. Verlaet, Annelies A., Daniela B. Noriega, Nina Hermans, and Huub F. Savelkoul. "Nutrition, Immunological Mechanisms and Dietary Immunomodulation in ADHD." *European Child & Adolescent Psychiatry* 23, no. 7 (2014), 519-529.

40. Verrotti, A., A. M. Tocco, C. Salladini, G. Latini, and F. Chiarelli. "Human Photosensitivity: From Pathophysiology to Treatment." *European Journal of Neurology* 12, no. 11 (2005), 828-841.

41. Weigal, George, and Kenneth F. Casey. *Striking Back!: The Trigeminal Neuralgia and Face Pain Handbook*. Gainesville, FL: TNA Facial Pain Association, 2004.

Publications from Association for Comprehensive NeuroTherapy

Available on Amazon.com and in our store: *Latitudes.org/store*

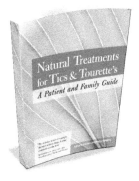

Natural Treatments for Tics & Tourette's: A Patient and Family Guide *by Sheila Rogers DeMare*

Tics and Tourette syndrome can often be treated naturally—without drugs or medications. Our bestselling book has 360 pages of helpful information. Join thousands of other families who have learned ways to eliminate or reduce their tics by using this book.

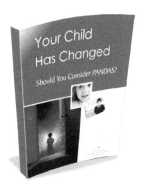

Your Child Has Changed: Should You Consider PANDAS? *by Laura Matheos with Sheila R DeMare*

Do you see dramatic changes in your child? Perhaps signs of separation anxiety, hyperactivity, OCD, tics or abnormal movements? Do you notice rapid mood swings, more frequent trips to the bathroom, or a sudden onset of anorexia? Any number of these can be symptoms of PANDAS. Written especially for parents, this eBook offers an understanding of what PANDAS is and is not, and how to find help.

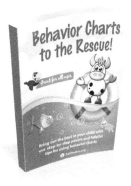

Behavior Charts to the Rescue! *By Mona Wimmer with Sheila Rogers DeMare*

For parents and teachers: This easy-to-read eBook will teach you how to select the best behavior charts to use, how to decide on the most appropriate low-cost rewards, what steps ensure your child or student's participation, and how to troubleshoot different scenarios as you help your child or student.

CPSIA information can be obtained
at www.ICGtesting.com
Printed in the USA
LVHW022249271018
595069LV00003B/14/P